THE PHILOSOPHY OF MATHEMATICS AND NATURAL LAWS

Dedicated to

Sir William Rowan Hamilton MRIA
1805–1865
Professor of Astronomy, Trinity College, Dublin
Astronomer Royal of Ireland

and

Sir Edmund Whittaker FRS
1873–1956
Astronomer Royal of Ireland
Professor of Mathematics,
University of Edinburgh

The Philosophy of Mathematics and Natural Laws

Another Copernican Revolution

NOEL CURRAN

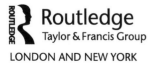
Routledge
Taylor & Francis Group

LONDON AND NEW YORK

First published 1997 by Ashgate Publishing

Reissued 2018 by Routledge
2 Park Square, Milton Park, Abingdon, Oxon, OX14 4RN
711 Third Avenue, New York, NY I 0017, USA

Routledge is an imprint of the Taylor & Francis Group, an informa business

Publisher's Note
The publisher has gone to great lengths to ensure the quality of this reprint but points out that some imperfections in the original copies may be apparent.

Disclaimer
The publisher has made every effort to trace copyright holders and welcomes correspondence from those they have been unable to contact.

A Library of Congress record exists under LC control number: 97073212

Typeset by Breeze Limited, Manchester.

ISBN 13: 978-1-138-33783-1 (hbk)
ISBN 13: 978-1-138-33784-8 (pbk)
ISBN 13: 978-0-429-44211-7 (ebk)

Contents

Preface   vii

Prolegomenon
Frege – the theory of judgement   1

1   Introduction   16

2   The concept of number   30

3   Number systems   35

4   Algebra – the science of pure time   55

5   Geometry   73

6   Measurement and numbers   95

7   Quaternions versus vector analysis   120

8   The unification of physics   136

    Section 1   The laws of nature   137

    Section 2   The arrow of time   139

Section 3   Einstein's special theory of relativity   142

Section 4   Einstein's general theory of relativity,
            theory of gravitation   155

Section 5   Quantum theory   157

Section 6   Cosmology – the Big Bang and the expansion
            of the universe   166

Section 7   The philosophy of science – especially the
            philosophy of mathematics and its
            applications to nature   169

Section 8   The relation between science and religion – the
            existence of a God or no God   177

References   191

Bibliography   199

Index   203

Preface

This book is a sequel to my first book, *The Logical Universe: The Real Universe*, published in 1994. That book is an account of the philosophy of science – the science of physics. There is a section on the philosophy of mathematics, and the last section is on natural theology, on the problem of the existence of God. The title of this book is modelled on Herman Weyl's *The Philosophy of Mathematics and Natural Science*. The expression 'Natural Science' was changed to 'Natural Laws' as being more appropriate. The book is dedicated to Sir William Rowan Hamilton and Sir Edmund Whittaker, as was the first book. The story of my scientific and philosophical studies is rather remarkable, going back for 60 years. I read some philosophy of science even as a student of medicine. After graduating I studied psychiatry and eventually became a consultant psychiatrist. I have now been retired for some years. My studies included Aristotle, St Thomas Aquinas, Kant and the moderns Husserl, Frege, Wittgenstein, Ayer and Heidegger. In the philosophy of science I am especially indebted to the works of Stephen Hawking, Roger Penrose, Paul Davies and John Barrow. Pais' biography of Einstein was particularly useful. I studied numerous books on time – the most important being Whitrow's work. Several books on time have been published since 1994, the most valuable being Paul Davies' *About Time* (1995), with its subtitle *Einstein's Unfinished Revolution*.

In the philosophy of mathematics I have made no use of axiomatic set theory. My philosophy of mathematics is based on Hamilton's ideas about the ordinal character of numbers, the real numbers, measure numbers, the scalar numbers and the extension to vectors. The final extension is to Hamilton's quaternions. I interpreted this algebra as comprising the mathematics of spin, or intrinsic angular momentum. This led me to a new theory of space–time or, more properly, time–space. This theory is based on the motion of spin, and not on the motion of translation as in Einstein's special theory of relativity. The motion of spin is absolute and requires no frame of reference or coordinates for its description. In the quadruple formula of quaternions the first symbol represents time, the other three represent the axes of a body subject to spin. The first symbol is a scalar number, a real number, and the time which it represents extends back into the past either to infinity or with a beginning. If it is assumed that time had a beginning then time would have an arrow, be asymmetric and, in the most correct terminology, be anisotropic, i.e. not the same in each direction.

The problem of the arrow of time is the most central and fundamental in the whole of physics. There is an arrow of time in living things and in human experience, but it is absent in the special and general theories of relativity – i.e. in gravitation theory – and in quantum theory. With the introduction of an arrow of time in my theory of time–space based on spin – and in consequence of a beginning of time – the concept of a flow of time is restored to physics. The explanation of gravitation is now the flow of time in one direction – the arrow of time. Non-Euclidean geometry, based on curved space, due to the presence of mass is no longer required, and space remains Euclidean. This is in effect another Copernican Revolution in three respects: absolute time is restored; time has an arrow, is asymmetrical and anisotropic; and thirdly, the whole theory is based on the motion of spin, which is more fundamental than the motion of translation.

The laws of nature, e.g. the conservation laws and the constancy of the speed of light, are as they are in consequence of the absence of an arrow of time. This is a consequence of the perceived wisdom that there is no beginning of time, which is seen as extending to infinity in the past. There is no expansion of the universe or a Big Bang to explain the beginning of time. My explanation for the beginning of time and an arrow of time is the creation of the universe by God at the beginning of time. The present laws of physics, in contrast, are based on the premise that there is no God. Atheist scientists say there is a conflict between science and religion, that science is right and religion is wrong, and that there is no God. His existence is not necessary as an explanation for any phenomenon in physics. I agree that the atheists are correct for the present state of physics. But there is no arrow of time in gravitation theory and quantum theory, and the two theories have not yet been unified successfully in spite of every effort being made to achieve this. I agree also that there is a conflict between science and religion, but I reverse the atheists' conclusion: in my view, science is wrong or incomplete, and religion is right – God created the universe at the beginning of time. In consequence of the beginning of time there is an arrow in physics, with all the changes that the introduction of such a concept produces.

Gravitation is thus a consequence of the flow of time in one direction – the arrow of time. God is not the God of the gaps but the God of gravitation. The introduction of an arrow of time into gravitation theory and quantum theory will result in changes in the laws of nature, including a change in the speed of light with the progression of time. This will open the way to a complete and general unification of these two fundamental branches of physics. Our explanation of gravitation now moves from one derived from geometry to one based on a time which is asymmetrical, or more correctly anisotropic, i.e. not the same in each direction, forward and backward. There would then be no mismatch between the time of living beings and human experience and the time of physics. Paul Davies refers to 'Einstein's Unfinished Revolution', but what is needed is another revolution: a change from relative time without an arrow to absolute time with an arrow. This is what I hope I have provided in this book.

Finally, I wish to thank my typist Frank Ramtohul for all his patience and care.

Manchester
October 1996

Prolegomenon
Frege – the theory of judgement

We will first examine Frege's theory of judgement, using his famous paper *Über Sinn und Bedeutung*, published in 1892. We use the English translation of the paper by Max Black as published in *Translations from the philosophical writings of Gottlob Frege* by Peter Geach and Max Black (1960). The paper translates as 'On Sense and Reference'. The German word '*Sinn*' can also be given as 'meaning', which I think is preferable. The translation of the word '*Bedeutung*' is confusing as the ordinary translation is 'meaning', but Frege is using it in a special way as 'reference': what a word, proper name or expression stands for. Therefore the translation of Frege's paper will be 'On Meaning and Reference'. The very first sentences of the paper state the main problem: 'Equality gives rise to challenging questions which are not altogether easy to answer. Is it a relation? A relation between objects, or between names or signs of objects? In my *Begriffsschrift* I assume the latter.'[1] In a footnote Frege states that equality means the same as identity. He gives two examples of equations expressing identity: $a = a$ and $a = b$. To clarify the use of the words judgement, proposition and sentence, I use judgement to mean a mental act or experience, proposition its verbal expression in spoken language, i.e. an auditory phenomenon, and sentence as the written expression of the judgement, i.e. a visual phenomenon. The sentence can be written or printed on paper, chalked on a blackboard, cut out in stone or illuminated in neon lights, etc. The distinction between meaning and reference can best be explained in a series of examples beginning with Frege's own first example, of the 'evening star' and the 'morning star'. These are best displayed as formulas by writing the expressions or proper names on the left-hand side with arrows to indicate the references.

1

In Frege's example, there are two different expressions with the same reference – i.e. two different meanings with the same reference:

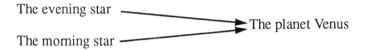

The evening star

The morning star

The planet Venus

Husserl in his first Logical Investigation, 'Expression and Meaning', is dealing with the same problem as Frege. In Section 12 he states: 'Names offer the plainest example of the separation of meaning from the relation to objects, this relation being in their case usually spoken of as "naming". Two names can differ in meaning but can have the same object, e.g.

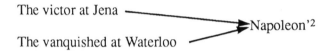

The victor at Jena

The vanquished at Waterloo

Napoleon'[2]

Frege's paper was well known to Husserl, and was in fact given as a reference in a footnote in Section 15 of the same Investigation.[3] It is worth noting that Husserl made no use of the second part of Frege's paper – on the theory of truth-functions – in the rest of his *Logical Investigations*.

The next example is of the distinction using proper names, or rather a proper name and a pseudonym:

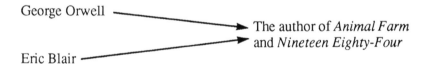

George Orwell

Eric Blair

The author of *Animal Farm* and *Nineteen Eighty-Four*

The next example is the list of seven honorary titles included in the litany of the Blessed Virgin Mary:

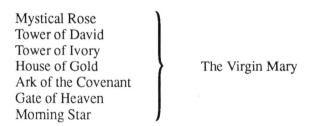

Mystical Rose
Tower of David
Tower of Ivory
House of Gold
Ark of the Covenant
Gate of Heaven
Morning Star

The Virgin Mary

Most people using or reciting this litany would not know the meaning of these titles or metaphors, but they naturally know the reference of the titles. It is an odd coincidence that the last expression, 'Morning Star', is used by Frege in his principal example.

The distinction between meaning and reference can be used to give some understanding of the Christian doctrine of the Trinity:

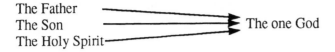

The Father
The Son   The one God
The Holy Spirit

The three persons of the Trinity have different meanings but the same reference – the one God. We now turn to the use of the distinction of meaning and reference in mathematics:

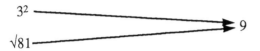

3^2

$\sqrt{81}$ 9

This can be expressed as an equation: $3^2 = \sqrt{81}$. This is a judgement or proposition of identity or equality. It is a judgement with one reference, the True.

Another example:

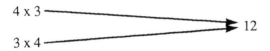

4×3

3×4 12

This again can be expressed as an equation: $4 \times 3 = 3 \times 4$. This multiplication is now expressed in symbolic form:

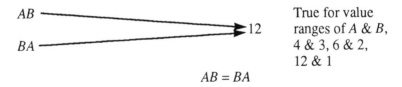

AB True for value
                          12   ranges of A & B,
BA 4 & 3, 6 & 2,
                                        12 & 1

$$AB = BA$$

This is the commutative law of multiplication – the order of the symbols makes no difference. $AB = BA$ – this judgement is true for all values of A and B.

If two expressions – e.g. the morning star and the evening star – have the same reference they are identical, they have equality, therefore they can be expressed as a judgement or proposition.

The morning star is the same as the evening star. This is a judgement with one reference, the True. Let us return to the mathematical examples:

$$3^2 = \sqrt{81}$$
$$AB = BA$$

These are analytical a priori judgements – in Kant's term they are apodeictic judgements, they are necessarily true. An axiom is a judgement with one reference, the true. This is the basis of Aristotle's demonstrative premise (apodeiktike protasis), an essential requirement for proof theory, or formal logic. Quoting from the first page of W. and M. Kneales' *The Development of Logic*:

> It is those types of discourse or inquiry in which *Proof* is sought or demanded that naturally give rise to logical investigation; for to prove a proposition is to infer its validity from true premises. The conditions of proof are two; true premises, or starting points, and valid arguments.[4]

The subject of the first section of the first chapter of the Kneales' book is the notion (concept) of validity. This concept is based on necessary truths – i.e. axioms – and is also used by Husserl in his *Ideas I*:

> The logical propositions to which it might find occasion to refer would thus throughout be logical *axioms* such as the principle of contradiction, whose universal and absolute validity, however, it could make transparent by the help of examples taken from the data of its own domain.[5]

Heidegger has a brief reference to validity in Section 33 of his *Being and Time*. He says that there is prevalent today a theory of 'judgement' which is oriented to the phenomenon of 'validity' – in German *Geltung*. He speaks of the very questionable character of the phenomenon of validity. Since the time of Lotze people have been calling it a 'primal phenomenon'. Heidegger then gives his considered opinion in one sentence:

> In the first place, validity is viewed as *'form of actuality'* which goes with the content of the judgement, in so far as that content remains unchanged as opposed to the changeable 'psychical' process of judgement.[6]

The concept of the validity of judgements is related not to the concept of the judgement but to its form, namely a judgement which has one reference – the True. These are judgements of identity or equality – they are true of necessity, i.e. they are valid judgements, judgements which have one reference. The true judgements are axioms – they are the foundation of axiomatic theory. Frege summarises what can be called the first part of his paper:

> To make short and exact expressions possible, let the following phraseology be established: A proper name (word, sign, sign combination, expression) expresses its sense, stands for or designates its reference. By means of a sign we express its sense and designate its reference.[7]

4

It is rather odd calling any expression or sign combination a 'proper name', and that term need not be used. One can hardly call $\sqrt{81}$ a 'proper name'.

The first part of Frege's paper is thus a theory of expression and meaning, to use the language of Husserl's First Logical Investigation. Two or more different expressions can have the same reference: therefore the expressions are equal to each other. This can be formulated as a judgement, proposition or sentence of equality or identity – i.e. a judgement with one reference, the true.

At the beginning of the second part of his paper, Frege says:

> So far we have considered the sense and reference only of such expressions, words or signs as we have called proper names. We now inquire concerning the sense and reference for an entire declarative sentence.[8]

But the first part of Frege's paper can also be formulated as an entire declarative sentence, i.e. a proposition or judgement as already described. Frege then gives his theory of truth values in three sentences:

> We are therefore driven into accepting the truth value of a sentence as constituting its reference. By the truth value of a sentence I understand the circumstance that it is true or false. There are no further truth values. For brevity I call the one the True the other the False. Every declarative sentence concerned with the reference of its words is therefore to be regarded as a proper name, and its reference, if it has one, is either the True or the False.[9]

A declarative sentence is a proposition, a judgement. There is now no need for us to use the unfamiliar term 'proper name' any longer. In this theory a judgement has two references – the True and the False – what is the case and what is not the case. The reference of the judgement is two states of affairs divided by a negation. The following are some examples:

> The red book is on the table
> The red book is not on the table.

In the entrance hall of hospitals there is usually a notice board indicating the presence or absence of the doctors. Wittgenstein gives the example of a similar notice board for students on the staircases of Oxford colleges. Dr Brown is *IN*. Dr Brown is *OUT*. From mathematics, $x^2 = 9$. This is true for values of $x + 3$ and -3 but false for all other values of x. The essence of a judgement is to be true or false, to have two references – the True and the False. For idealist logicians such as Bradley, judgements are essentially true or false. This is pointed out by Gilbert Ryle in his introduction to *The Revolution in Philosophy*:

> Next both [Frege and Bradley] saw that it is not extrinsic but intrinsic to a thought to be true or false, or to have 'objective reference'. When I judge, I judge that

something is the case. If it is not the case, then I have misjudged; and the allegation that I have misjudged implies that something else is the case. In saying what we think, we do not just signal what is going on in our heads, we describe or else we mis-describe reality.[10]

Wittgenstein's picture theory in the *Tractatus* is the theory of judgement with two references, the True and the False:

A picture depicts reality by representing a possibility of existence and non-existence of states of affairs.[11]

and again:

A proposition must restrict reality to two alternatives: YES or NO.[12]

Elizabeth Anscombe describes the relationship between Frege's theory of truth-function and Wittgenstein's picture theory with greatest clarity:

Indeed, we should not regard Wittgenstein's theory of the proposition as a *synthesis* of a picture theory and the theory of truth-functions; his picture theory and the theory of truth-functions are one and the same. Every genuine proposition picks out certain existences and non-existences of states of affairs, as a range within which the actual existences and non-existences of states of affairs are to fall. Something with the appearance of a proposition, but which does not do this, cannot really be saying anything, it is not a description of any reality.[13]

It is in fact not a question of the *appearance* of a proposition which does not do this, but a proposition with one reference only – the True – a theory of equality, a theory of identity, an apodeictic proposition. The distinction between judgements with one reference, the True, and judgements with two references, the True and the False, is of course nothing new – it was made very clearly by Aristotle, to quote from the Kneales' book on *The Development of Logic*:

It is not easy to tell how soon it was realised that the two conditions are independent, but it was perfectly clear to Aristotle when he drew the distinction between apodeictic and dialectical reasoning in the *Topics* and again in the *Prior Analytics*. The latter is worth quoting in full because it throws light on the content in which the distinction was first drawn.

The demonstrative premise (apodeiktike protasis) differs from the dialectical because the demonstrative is the assumption of one of a pair of contradictory propositions (for the man who demonstrates assumes something and does not ask a question), but the dialectical premise is a question as to which of two contra-dictions is true.[14]

The demonstrative premise is true and necessary – a judgement with one reference, the True. This is formal logic – axiomatic theory, a theory of proof. Formal logic is concerned with principles of valid inference – a theory of validity.

By contrast, dialectical logic holds that, for a judgement to have meaning in the fullest sense, it must have two references, the True and the False. There are no axioms. The most fundamental assumptions are falsified, i.e. negated. A significant proposition is one which can be falsified. Abelard developed and used dialectical logic in the twelfth century in his work *Sic Et Non*, derived from Aristotle's *Topics*. This was the basis of the scholastic method used by St Thomas Aquinas in the thirteenth century. Every article in *Summa Theologica* has three parts: the first contains all the objections – the falsification of the doctrine under discussion – then follows the body of the article giving the true account as he understands it, and the third part is a reply to each of the objections in the first part. This is in effect the application of dialectical logic, not an axiomatic method. Dialectical logic is a theory of meaning. Formal logic is a theory of validity and proof.

Frege in his introduction to his *Foundations of Arithmetic* describes three fundamental principles which he proposes to use. The second is the context principle, namely 'never to ask for the meaning of a word in isolation, but only in the context of a proposition'. This was published in 1884, well before *On Meaning and Reference*. The first part of the latter paper is in effect a theory of the judgement or proposition with only one reference, the True – a theory of identity, a theory of equality. The second part of the paper is the theory of truth-functions. The judgements or propositions here have two references – the True and the False. This is a theory of difference, a theory of meaning. In each case the form of the judgement is considered. But the content of the judgement must also be considered. The examples already given are trivial contingent facts – the red book is on the table, the red book is not on the table. We must apply to mathematics the theory of dialectical logic – that is, judgements with the two references, the True and the False, i.e. two states of affairs divided by a negation. In the commutative law of multiplication $AB = BA$; the order makes no difference – i.e. commutative algebra. But non-commutative algebras have been developed, the first one being Hamilton's quaternions, where $AB \neq BA$; the order of multiplication here does make a difference: $AB = -BA$. The numbers are not cardinal numbers, they are vectors in three dimensions. Matrix algebra developed by Cayley is also non-commutative. It is logically impossible to include these algebras in formal logic, where judgements have only one reference, the True – i.e. a theory of identity or equality. In quantum mechanics, the linear operators which correspond to the dynamical variables are subject to an algebra in which the commutative axiom of multiplication does not hold. In other words the equations of motion do not commute. In classical mechanics the equations of motion do commute. You therefore have in dynamics two states of affairs which are contradictory, i.e. divided by a negation – namely the dynamical operators commute and do not commute, i.e. what is the case and what is not the case. These contradictory theories, one of which is the foundation of classical mechanics and the other the fundamental principle of quantum mechanics, cannot be incorporated in a system of formal logic. In formal logic the judgements or propositions have only one reference, the True – it is a theory of identity or equality as described in the first part of Frege's paper. But both these contradictory theories can be accommodated in dialectical logic because the judgements or propositions have two references, the True and the False – what is the case and what is not the case – and can thus use commutative and non-commutative algebra. This problem cannot be solved by the use of the principle of value-ranges in formal logic:

> More important than these is a remark in the lecture *Function and Begriff* of 1891. In that lecture, Frege explained the changes in his formal and philosophical logic that he had made during the silent years that separated his early from his middle period. In particular he explained the introduction into his formal logic of the new notion of a value-range, where a value-range is to function as a class is to a concept.[15]

The following example will show the use of value-ranges: $x^2 = 9$. This is true for the value if $x = +3$ and -3 and false for all other values of x. In commutative algebra $AB = BA$ – the order of multiplication makes no difference. In non-commutative algebra $AB \neq BA$ the value, i.e. the value-ranges are the same for the commutative and non-commutative algebras. The reason for the non-identity in non-commutative algebra is that the *order* of multiplication makes a difference. This state of affairs is impossible in formal logic, where the proposition has only one reference, the True – i.e. an analytic a priori proposition which is necessarily true and cannot be contradicted. But in dialectical logic the two states of affairs – commutative and non-commutative multiplication – can both be included because the proposition has two references, the True and the False. The commutative law of multiplication cannot be an axiom, so the problem of the proof of the law is no longer required.

Exactly the same situation arises with the axioms of Euclidean geometry, especially with the parallel axiom – its contradictory gives various types of non-Euclidean geometry.

The difference between Euclidean and non-Euclidean geometry can be expressed in the form of equation – i.e. a proposition of equality. For Euclidean geometry the internal angles of a triangle are equal to 180°. For non-Euclidean geometry the internal angles of a triangle are not equal to 180°; they are greater than or less than 180°, depending on whether the curvature is positive or negative (the Euclidean geometry has zero curvature, i.e. space is flat). This can be expressed more briefly in symbolic form:

Euclidean geometry	Non-Euclidean geometry
angles of $\Delta = 180°$	angles of $\Delta \neq 180°$; > or < 180°

The existence of non-Euclidean geometry was of course well known to Frege. The judgements in the logic of arithmetic are analytic a priori, i.e. true necessarily. As the axioms of Euclidean geometry can be contradicted Frege could not include geometry in his philosophy of mathematics. This problem is described in some detail in Section 14 of his *Grundlagen* and is quoted in full in Dummett's book *Frege – Philosophy of Mathematics*. Part of the quotation is as follows:

> For conceptual thought we can always assume the opposite of this or that geometrical axiom, without involving ourselves in any self-contradictions when we draw deductions conflicting with intuition such as these. This possibility shows that the axioms of geometry are independent of one another and of the fundamental laws of logic, and are therefore synthetic. Can one say the same of the fundamental principles of the science of number? Does not everything collapse in confusion when we try denying one of them?[16]

At the end of the quotation from Frege Dummett comments:

> That the axioms of geometry can be denied without contradiction does not prove that they are synthetic; it is what is meant by saying that they are synthetic.

This is not the correct interpretation of synthetic a priori judgements, as the term is used by Kant. These are the same as analytic judgements in that they are necessary. They are also judgements with one reference – this is clearly stated by Kant with reference to natural science in his *Prolegomena to any Future Metaphysics*:

> Natural Science (Physica) contains in itself synthetic judgements a priori as principles. I will only cite a few propositions: that in all changes in the corporeal world the quantity of matter remains unchanged, or that in all communication of movement action and reaction must always be equal. Both, it is clear, are not only necessary and a priori in origin, but also synthetic.[17]

Therefore Kant's synthetic a priori judgements cannot be contradicted; they are the same as the analytic a priori judgements in that they have only one reference – the True. In Kant's example from physics the conservation laws – for example of matter (mass) – are true necessarily, they are axioms.

The axioms of Euclidean and non-Euclidean geometry cannot be included in the fundamental laws of formal logic. But, just as was the case with commutative and non-commutative algebra, Euclidean and non-Euclidean geometry can be included in dialectical logic. The problem of trying to prove the parallel axiom for Euclidean geometry does not arise. The problem is one of the meaning of Euclidean and non-Euclidean. Euclidean geometry means there is zero curvature of space, and space can be infinite in extension. For non-Euclidean geometry space is curved and finite but unbounded. Both states of affairs can be accepted in dialectical logic.

Frege in the quotation above refers to the fundamental principles of the science of number, and states that everything collapses in confusion when we try denying one of them. In Section 12 of the *Grundlagen* he mentions the commutative and associative laws of addition, but he does not mention one of the most fundamental operations in mathematics, namely multiplication. There are commutative and non-commutative algebras – two different laws of multiplication which are contradictory. Formal logic cannot account for both; instead, dialectical logic must be used.

Up to now we have only used examples from mathematics and physics. We now show the use of dialectical logic in a problem of the greatest importance and generality, namely the duration of time and whether time has a beginning, or extends to infinity in the past. We have two states of affairs: time has a beginning and time has no beginning. These states of affairs are contradictory: they represent what is the case and what is not the case. These opposed conditions cannot be accounted for in formal logic, which depends on analytic judgements which are true necessarily. Exactly the same situation applies to the problem of the arrow of time – i.e. time direction, or in German *Zeitrichtung* – or no arrow of time: again they are contradictory states of affairs. If time has no beginning is an axiom, the possibility of its having a beginning is logically impossible. If time has no arrow, no characteristic of direction – i.e. forward and backward are no different – is an axiom, then the possibility of time having an arrow or direction is also logically impossible. But with dialectical logic both states of affairs are possible and any physical consequence of the two states of affairs can be considered.

Frege's paper on meaning and reference is concerned primarily with the form of the judgement and not with the content of the judgement; at least, that is its most important aspect. The judgement has two forms. The first part of Frege's paper is on the judgement with one reference – i.e. a theory of identity or equality – the one reference is the True. Strictly speaking, Frege was concerned with the meaning and reference of expressions, but in fact these can be put in the form of a declarative sentence, i.e. a judgement or proposition.

The second part of Frege's paper is on declarative sentences, i.e. judgements which have two references – the True and the False, what is the case and what is not the case. The problem of the form and content of judgements can be elucidated by Husserl's theory of intentionality. All conscious experience is of something, i.e. a content, but the form of the experience also has to be considered – this is in Husserl's terminology the noetic and noematic aspect of the experience. The noetic is the form or quality of the experience; the noematic is the content of the experience. Husserl devotes 100 pages to this important distinction – Sections 87 to 127 – in Boyce Gibson's English translation of *Ideas – General Introduction to Pure Phenomenology* (1931). An example from the auditory phenomenon of spoken language will show the distinction very clearly. You can have the same words – the same content – spoken by different people; it could be a male voice, a female voice, spoken with different accents, fast or slow, with different pitches, a bass voice, soprano or falsetto. The distinction is so subtle that individual voices can be recognised. This is the noetic aspect of the experience. The same distinction is shown when one hears music played. The same melody – the same content, or noema – but with different instruments has different qualities of sound, e.g. with a piano, violin, clarinet, oboes, etc. The notes of the melody are the same – i.e. it has the same noema or content – but the noesis, i.e. the form or quality, is different. This difference can easily be recognised by anyone with a modest knowledge of music. With the experience of judgements the same distinctions apply. The noesis is the form of the judgements, of which there are two – the judgement with one reference, the True, as in the first part of Frege's paper, and the judgement with two references, the True and the False, as in the second part of his paper. This is the most important contribution of Frege to the theory of logic. The content of the judgements is also of importance – the noema, the noematic aspect. Such judgements can often be trivial and contingent, e.g. the red book is on the table or in nursery language the cat is on the mat, and the real value of the distinction only comes with important and highly generalised concepts, such as time with a beginning or no beginning, and time with an arrow or no arrow. In mathematics the same distinction is applied to judgements involved in commutative and non-commutative multiplication. These distinctions can be expressed in simple symbolic form:

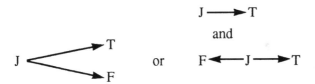

In the last example the judgement can be said to have two poles – the judgements are polar opposites. This term is used by Frege in his article on negation:

> This judging and negating look like a pair of polar opposites, which being a pair are coordinate, a pair comparable e.g. to oxidation and reduction in chemistry.[18]

He frequently refers to the polar opposite of judging. An excellent example of polar opposites in mathematics is commutative and non-commutative multiplication. Analogical language does not apply to this distinction. In analogical language there is something which is partly the same and partly different; there is an element of proportion between two concepts. In polar opposites there is no proportion – the two concepts are contradictory. This is impossible in analytical judgements, which have only one reference, the True; it is only possible when the judgement has two references, the True and the False, i.e. in dialectical logic.

In the introduction to the *Grundlagen* Frege says he has kept to three fundamental principles. The second one, as we have seen, is 'never to ask for the meaning of a word in isolation, but only in the context of a proposition'. This principle is used in the first part of his paper – the proposition has one reference, the True. Different words or expressions can have the same reference. But the same words or expressions often have different meanings. This is Wittgenstein's important dictum, as described in his *Philosophical Investigations*: 'the meaning of a word is its use in the language'.

The expression – i.e. the words – 'morning star' can have three different meanings:

1 The planet Venus.
2 An honorary title – e.g. the metaphorical title of the Blessed Virgin Mary.
3 The name of the communist daily newspaper in England.

In this example it would be difficult to find such diverse meanings for the same expression. Another example from Wittgenstein's *Brown Book* is 'bank', which could mean a river bank or the place for your money. The author remarks that children find it very difficult to grasp that the same word can have different meanings.

The most important word in the philosophy of mathematics is 'number'. What is the meaning of 'number'? Applying Wittgenstein's dictum that the meaning of a word is its use in the language, the word 'number' has two quite distinct uses, one for counting particular individual objects – cardinal numbers – and the other for measurement – the real numbers. There are thus different uses or applications of numbers. In Volume II, Section 157 of the *Grundgesetze* Frege says:

> Since cardinal numbers (*Anzahlen*) are not ratios we have to distinguish them from the positive whole numbers. It is therefore not possible to extend the domain of cardinal numbers to that of the real numbers; they are completely disjoint domains. The cardinal numbers answer the question, How many objects of a given kind are there? Whereas the real numbers can be regarded as measurement numbers, which state how large a quantity is as compared with a unit quantity.[19]

The operation of counting applies to both types of numbers. The farmer counts the number of sheep in his flock, and children count marbles and bricks in the kindergarten. Measure numbers are also counted. You count the number of metres in a piece of cloth, and the minutes, hours, days etc. are counted. As the two uses of the concept of number are so different – in Frege's words they are 'completely disjoint domains' – why not base the philosophy of mathematics on the real numbers, i.e. measure numbers only, without making any use of the cardinal numbers? The farmers and the children can keep the cardinal numbers for their own use. The measure numbers – the real numbers – are fundamental for the physical sciences, including astronomy. One of the most fundamental reference books in science, the *Astronomical Almanac*, has about 500 pages, each containing many thousands of measure numbers. There are nine planets – a cardinal number – but nowhere in the book is this fact actually stated, and no use is made of cardinal numbers.

The fact that the same word or expression can have different meanings is not included in Frege's context principle – as he says, we should ask for the meaning of a word only in the context of a proposition. The fact that the same word can have different meanings is thus completely ignored in that principle. The difference between the first part of Frege's paper and Wittgenstein's dictum about the meaning of words can be expressed very briefly:

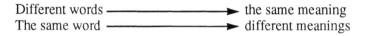

Different words ⟶ the same meaning
The same word ⟶ different meanings

We must next consider the difference between 'nonsense' and 'meaning-less', two words which of necessity are quite different from one another in their apperance and etymology, since to say that something is 'non-meaning' or 'unmeaning' is not correct use of English. In German, where the two terms are derived from the same noun *Sinn*, signifying sense or meaning, the expressions are *unsinn* – nonsense – and *sinnlos* – meaningless. If I say that my aunt Jemima is a right-angled triangle that is nonsense – *unsinn*; if I say that there are fairies at the bottom of my garden that is meaningless – *sinnlos*. The latter proposition has no meaning; it is meaningless because there are no empirical facts for or against the existence of fairies in the garden. But it is not nonsense. A child would have no difficulty in drawing a fairy using her imagination, i.e. as a work of fiction. These are trivial examples of the distinction, but when it is applied to problems of the greatest generality – e.g. the existence or non-existence of God – it is most important to understand the distinction correctly. The following is a quotation from Ayer's *Language, Truth and Logic* on this distinction as applied to the existence of God:

> And our view that all utterances about the nature of God are nonsensical, so far from being identical with, or even lending any support to, either of these familiar contentions is actually incompatible with them.[20]

In this sentence Ayer is using the wrong language; instead of 'nonsensical' he should have said 'without meaning' – 'meaningless'. In German it should be *sinnlos*, not *unsinn*. His very next sentence gives the correct interpretation of this distinction:

> For if the assertion that there is a god is nonsensical, then the atheist assertion that there is no god is equally nonsensical, since it is only a significant proposition that can be significantly contradicted.

In other words, a significant proposition is one which has two references, the True and the False – what is the case and what is not the case. This is the theme of the second part of Frege's paper and of Wittgenstein's picture theory of language. It is very different from assertions which are nonsense – these have no empirical reference whatsoever. Axioms are propositions which have only one reference, the True; their negation by definition is non-existent. Therefore axioms are not meaningful in the same way as propositions which can be contradicted – i.e. which have two references, the True and the False.

In the Aristotelian and Ptolemaic system of the cosmos, the earth was the centre of the universe and at rest in two respects: there was no motion of translation and no intrinsic spin. The system had three axioms:

1 The apparent motion of the stars and sun were due to the rotation of the celestial sphere.
2 The rate of rotation of this sphere was constant, which provided the perfect measure of time.
3 The universe was eternal.

The Copernican Revolution was the rejection of the first axiom. If the axiomatic system of the Ptolemaic universe had been retained there would have been no Copernican Revolution. David Hilbert at the International Mathematical Congress in 1900 listed 23 problems for solution in the future. The sixth problem was to axiomatise mathematical physics. If mathematics was based on an axiomatic system, why not physics also? But an axiomatic basis for mathematics cannot account for non-commutative algebra, where equations are equal and not equal. The non-equality is due not to the use of value-ranges: the values of the numbers remain the same, the only difference is in the order of the numbers. In classical mechanics the equations of motion are equal, they commute. But in quantum mechanics non-commutative algebra is used, the equations are not equal, they do not commute. The order of the operators makes a difference. These different theories cannot be included in an axiomatic system of logic. They can only be accounted for by a dialectical logic, where the judgement has two references, the True and the False, two states of affairs which are contradictory. Dialectical logic concentrates one's attention on the meaning of the judgement and the truth. However, the full understanding and meaning of quantum mechanics is not yet accepted by all physicists. Wittgenstein emphasised that mathematics uses equations:

> It is the essential characteristic of mathematical method that it employs equations. Indeed it is a consequence of this method that every proposition of mathematics must be obviously true.[21]

Putting the problem in different language, the equations of mathematics are tautologies. As already explained there are important branches of mathematics where the equations are not equal – various types of non-commutative algebra such as quaternions and matrix algebra. The theory of equality – that judgements have only one reference, the True – is the first part of Frege's paper. This is the foundation of formal logic. But this logic cannot account for the contradictory state of affairs when the equations are not equal. For this state of affairs dialectical logic must be used.

To summarise my thesis on Frege's *On Meaning and Reference*, the paper is in two parts: the first on judgement with one reference – the True – the second on judgement with two references – the True and the False. Both parts are concerned with the form of the judgement, not the content, or, in Husserl's language of intentionality, the noetic aspect of the judgement, not the noematic aspect.

The differences between the two parts can be given in tabular form:

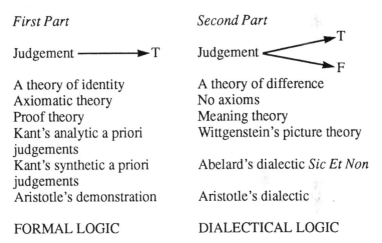

First Part	Second Part
Judgement ⟶ T	Judgement ⟨ T / F
A theory of identity	A theory of difference
Axiomatic theory	No axioms
Proof theory	Meaning theory
Kant's analytic a priori judgements	Wittgenstein's picture theory
Kant's synthetic a priori judgements	Abelard's dialectic *Sic Et Non*
Aristotle's demonstration	Aristotle's dialectic
FORMAL LOGIC	DIALECTICAL LOGIC

A judgement with one reference – the True – has validity. However, a judgement has meaning in the fullest sense only when it can be contradicted or negated, i.e. when it has two references – the True and the False – this is dialectical logic. Michael Dummett has often said that in any system of philosophy you must begin with the right logic. Dialectical logic, not formal logic, is the right logic, and it can be applied to the philosophy of mathematics and the philosophy of physics. Dialectical logic will provide the gateway to meaning and truth in these domains.

1 Introduction

The first problem to consider is how does one study the philosophy of mathematics. Is it necessary to be a professional mathematician to make a contribution or to understand what its philosophy is all about? The great names in the history of the subject, such as Husserl, Frege, Cantor, Peano, Hilbert, Whitehead and Russell, and in more modern times Gödel and Dummett, were all trained as mathematicians. The subject is usually called mathematical logic: therefore a general theory of logic is required, which is a fundamental part of the general subject of philosophy also. I think that a technical knowledge of mathematics is not essential for the philosophy of mathematics. All mathematical concepts can be expressed in language; thus, if a new concept is developed, a new language can be found to express it. A new word must be found for the new concept, usually from the Greek or Latin language. Therefore the study of the philosophy of mathematics can be an exercise in linguistic analysis. The fact that there are three schools of thought – the logicist, the formalist and the intuitionist – is sufficient evidence that the foundations of mathematics are not universally agreed. There is an interesting way of looking at the foundations of mathematics and comparing it with architecture. In constructing a building the foundations are laid first and the building is raised on top of that, reaching completion with the roof. In mathematics the procedure appears to be the reverse. There is an immense structure of mathematics built up over the centuries, but the very foundations of mathematics – what it really means – have not yet been provided.

In studying philosophy one must read the works of other writers, so as to understand their concepts on the subject. Yet there can be an overemphasis on this use of texts, and an almost endless series of comments on the texts can result, so much so that the fundamental problems of the subject are almost forgotten.

The fundamental concept of mathematics is that of number. Once that is established, one naturally has to use the texts of other people on the subject. One may agree or not agree with the concepts expressed in the texts of other philosophers, yet even when the views expressed in these works are the opposite of one's own ideas they can be most valuable in helping to find the truth of the matter. After all, there are only two possibilities. What is said in the text is either correct or incorrect, or, in the ideas used in our own theory of the philosophy of mathematics, what is the case and what is not the case.

But finally you must develop a complete and coherent account of the philosophy. Therefore I must develop my own philosophy of mathematics, which of course will agree or not agree with the views expressed in the texts of other mathematicians or philosophers of mathematics. I have noticed a remarkable fact about the general theories of philosophers or scientists as expounded in their texts. Even in a complete book on the subject, the fundamental or central ideas are often expressed somewhere in one paragraph and often even in one sentence. This is of course most helpful in using quotations from the texts, which can agree or not agree with one's own point of view.

Logic

Before one can begin a philosophy of mathematics it is essential to have a theory of logic. The foundation of any theory of logic is the judgement. For this purpose I propose to use the text of Frege's famous paper of 1892, *Über Sinn und Bedeutung*. This paper is considered so important that the October 1992 issue of the philosophy journal *Mind* was entirely devoted to it, to commemorate its centenary. I have written an article on the paper which was worked out a considerable time before I had read the issue in question. This article was sent to *Mind* in November 1992 but was not accepted for publication. The following is a brief summary of my paper on Frege's *Über Sinn und Bedeutung*. The standard translation of Frege's paper is *On Sense and Reference*, but I prefer to use a different translation, *On Meaning and Reference*. The paper is essentially in two parts.

The first part

In this, different expressions or words have the same reference.

Using a mathematical example:

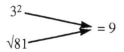

The two expressions have the same reference, namely the number 9. That is, the expressions are equal – it is a theory of identity. It is in effect a declarative sentence – a judgement with one reference, the True. This is what an axiom means: a judgement which is necessarily true; its negation is non-existent. These judgements are the same as Kant's analytic a priori judgements: they are true of necessity – if they are axioms. His synthetic a priori judgements are also true of necessity, i.e. axioms. In a paper I wrote showing that Kant's synthetic a priori judgements were true necessarily I gave a reference to his *Prolegomena to any Future Metaphysics*. But in Section 2 of the introduction to the *Critique of Pure Reason* Kant makes it very clear that it is the a priori character of the judgements, analytic and synthetic, which ensures that character of necessity, i.e. they are both axioms: judgements with one reference, the True:

> Now in the first place, if we have a proposition which contains the idea of necessity in its very conception, it is a judgement a priori; if moreover it is not derived from any other proposition, unless from one equally involving the idea of necessity, it is absolutely a priori.[1]

Husserl in Section 16 of *Ideas I* makes very clear and explicit reference to Kant's synthetic a priori judgements:

> If, despite notable differences in fundamental outlook which are not incompatible however with an inner affinity, one wishes to maintain approval of Kant's *Critique of the Reason*, one has only to interpret the regional axioms as synthetic cognitions a priori and we should then have as many irreducible classes of such forms of knowledge as there are regions.[2]

Cognitions are of course judgements. Husserl's interpretation of Kant's synthetic a priori judgements is perfectly correct. He calls them axioms. The regional axioms are to be used for different regions of knowledge, such as mathematics, physics, biology, etc.

The first part of Frege's paper is really a theory of judgements of identity – judgements which are true, which have one reference, the True.

Different words can have the same reference. Frege's first example is:

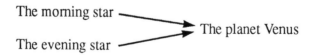

This can be expressed in very simple symbolic form:

In this part of Frege's paper he says that so far we have considered the meaning and reference of words or expressions. We now enquire concerning the meaning and reference of an entire declarative sentence. The declarative sentence is a judgement or proposition. But, as I explained in the previous chapter, the first part of Frege's paper is really a judgement – a declarative sentence of identity – with one reference, the True, i.e. an axiom. He then goes on to give an account of the truth value of a sentence. Every judgement is true or false. It states what is the case and what is not the case. The judgement has two references – the True and the False. The judgements are contradictory, they are divided by a negation. They are not now judgements of identity, but judgements of difference. However, to say that this is the essence of a judgement or that all judgements have two references – the True and the False – is not correct. There is an important exception. Some judgements have only one reference – the True – i.e. axioms. Judgements with two references – the True and the False – can be falsified. Judgements with only one reference – the True – i.e. axioms, cannot be falsified – their negation is non-existent.

The judgement with two references can be expressed very simply:

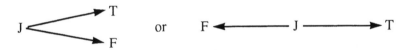

The second form of the judgement is expressed as two poles: the judgements are polar opposites. Two contradictory states of affairs – what is the case and what is not the case – are polar opposites. This is the use of polar language. It is different from analogical language, where two states of affairs are partly the same and partly different – i.e. there is a proportion between the two states of affairs. With polar language there is no proportion: the two states of affairs are contradictory, they are divided by a negation; that is, the judgement has two references, the True and the False.

To have meaning in the fullest sense, a judgement must have two references – the True and the False. It must be capable of verification and falsification. There must be a state of affairs corresponding to its being true and its being false. There are therefore two types of judgements:

1   Judgements with one reference, the True – i.e. axioms.
2   Judgements with two references, the True and the False.

In formal logic proof is a fundamental concept. For proof theory you require true premises, i.e. axioms and valid arguments. Axioms are judgements with one reference – the True – their negation by definition is impossible and non-existent. Judgements with two references – the True and the

False – have meaning. They have no axioms, for this is dialectical logic. Examples of judgements which are true and false can be very trivial: the red ball is on the table, it is not on the table. But when the distinction is applied to very general concepts such as whether space is flat or curved, time has a beginning or no beginning and even to whether there is a God or no God, problems of the most fundamental nature are involved. Equations in mathematics such as $7 + 5 = 12$ or $7 \times 5 = 5 \times 7$ have validity. Wittgenstein called them tautologies. They are of the same status as 'Bachelors are unmarried men.' He called them in his language *sinnlos* – i.e. meaningless – but they have validity.

In the two parts of Frege's paper we have been concerned with the meaning of judgements. The meaning of words or expressions without reference to judgements has not been considered. In the first part of his paper Frege stated that different words and expressions can have the same meaning or reference. We now consider the important distinction that the same word can have different meanings – i.e. the opposite state of affairs. This is Wittgenstein's famous dictum that the meaning of a word is its use in the language – implying that the same word can have different meanings or uses. Let us take as an example an expression from the first part of Frege's paper – the morning star. This has at least two meanings:

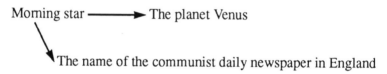

An important example very relevant to mathematics is the word 'number', e.g.

1 Cardinal numbers, the answer to the question how many objects of a given kind?
2 Real numbers, which are measurement numbers.

The following is a very brief list of some of the differences between formal logic and dialectical logic in tabular form:

Formal Logic	*Dialectical Logic*
Use of axioms	No axioms
A theory of identity	A theory of difference
A theory of proof	A theory of meaning
A theory of validity	

I now propose to give a brief account of axiomatic set theory.

Axiomatic set theory

I have made a list of 12 concepts involved in axiomatic set theory. This will obviously include the concept of a set and axioms and many other problems in the philosophy of mathematics. The basic concept is that of number – we begin with cardinal numbers.

1 Cardinal numbers and sets

The word is derived from the Latin *cardo* – a hinge. Everything hinges on it, meaning it is most important and fundamental, as Frege says. Cardinal numbers answer the question: how many objects of a given kind are there? The number of objects is the set or class. Numerous other words are used to describe the concept of a set of things: groups, aggregate, collection – 'collective' is the term used by Husserl. Cantor defined a set as a collection of definite well-distinguished objects for perception or thought – the elements of a set – gathered together into a whole! Examples could be four apples in a bowl, three coins in the fountain, the twelve apostles, six beans in a box. There are special words for a group or class of animals, for example a flock of sheep, a herd of cows. But it is not so easy to see how these set numbers apply to the natural physical world. There are, reasonably enough, a set or class of nine planets, the atomic number of an element, the number of electrons in each atom, and it seems reasonable to speak of a set, group or collection of animals of the same kind, such as five sheep, but is it a set if all five animals are different, e.g. one dog, one cat, one horse, one cow and one pig? The answer to this question has no relevance for mathematics or physics. One can consider a set of points along a line as also constituting a set, although this is unsatisfactory.

2 One-to-one correspondence

Two numbers are equal and therefore two sets are equal – if there is a one-to-one correspondence between them. Frege gives the well-known example of the knives and forks at a well-set dinner table. If there are twelve plates, each with one knife on the right and one fork on the left, it is not necessary to count them all separately. If you count the plates, then the number of knives and forks are the same: the numbers match or correspond or correlate. A shepherd who is not very bright is asked to count a large flock of sheep. He is given a box of pebbles and a bowl. The sheep are driven through a narrow gate, and he puts one pebble in the bowl for each sheep that passes through the gate. The number of pebbles in the bowl correlate, correspond or match the number of sheep in the flock. A more sophisticated method is often used to count the number of people attending meetings or on a train or perhaps at their church. A counting device is used – a button is pressed as each person enters and a number is indicated on a dial, the number increasing in sequence as the button is pressed. At the end the total can be read from the dial. That number will match or correlate with the number of people attending the meeting or on the train, etc. The two numbers are equal – a one-to-one correspondence has been established.

3 The problem of 0 and 1

If a cardinal number is the number of members, objects or individuals of a set, class or group, what is meant by a set, etc. with no members? This appears to be a contradiction. One can think of an example: there are no members of the class Chinese popes. But this is pure fiction – it corresponds to nothing in reality. The number 1 also presents a problem. If a set is defined as an aggregate, collection or plurality of objects or individuals, then if there is only one member in the group this also appears to be a contradiction. If someone said he was a stamp collector but had only one stamp, it would be considered ridiculous – a contradiction. What does the number 1 mean in the physical universe? It could mean one atom, one electron, one planet, one moon or perhaps one universe. But that is not of much value for developing mathematical physics.

4 Cardinal numbers and ordinal numbers

The series of natural numbers represented by the integers 0, 1, 2, 3, 4 . . . are obviously in an ordered sequence: they are ordinal numbers. Peano's axioms of number are set down very clearly; the first four are:

1   1 is a number.
2   The successor to any number is a number.
3   No two numbers have the same successor.
4   1 is not the successor of any number.

The number 0 was later placed at the beginning giving the sequence as above, i.e. 0, 1, 2, 3, 4 . . . But the cardinal numbers, the numbers of a set, class or group of individual members of the set, have no ordinal character.

The number of boys in a class is 20 – this is the cardinal number of the set. The ordinal character of that number is totally absent. An ordinal character can only be introduced by artificial means, for example by putting the boys in order of the marks they receive in an examination in some subject. If the subject of the examination was different, the order of the boys in each case would most likely be different too. The order following each of the different examinations is not permanent but variable and accidental. A permanent order could be given to the boys by using their date of birth or perhaps their height. Twenty good-quality golf balls or tennis balls in a box have no order whatsoever. There is no way of putting them in order since they are all the same size, weight and colour. Set numbers, i.e. cardinal numbers, have no order in themselves unless it is put there by special procedure. The numbers of the pages in a book are ordinal, as is the case with the numbers of the houses in a street, the numbers on car registration plates, the numbers on passports, all of which are ordinal. But these numbers lack the character of set except by accident. Since, as we have seen, cardinal numbers or set numbers have no intrinsic ordinal character unless it is put there by extrinsic procedure, it would seem obvious that ordinal numbers are more important and more fundamental than cardinal numbers. Russell, however, totally rejects this point of view:

> In counting it is necessary to take the objects counted in a certain order, as first, second, third etc., but order is not the essence of number; it is an irrelevant addition, an unnecessary complication from the logical point of view. The notion of similarity does not demand an order: for example, we saw that the number of husbands is the same as the number of wives, without having to establish an order of precedence among them.[3]

Of course he is thinking of set or class numbers, and he is quite correct that set numbers are not ordinal, that the ordinal character is absent. In comparing the identity of two set numbers which are in one-to-one correspondence, like the knives and forks in a correctly set dinner table in Frege's example or Russell's own example of the husband and wives, their ordinal character is completely unnecessary. Therefore the ordinal character of numbers is not essential to Russell because he is using the concept of sets. This is a most serious indictment of set theory. Should I go so far as to say it is a fatal indictment?

Later in the same work Russell again comments on the relative importance of cardinal and ordinal numbers:

> For these reasons, it was only gradually that the importance of cardinals in mathematical philosophy was recognised; the importance of ordinals, though by no means small, is distinctly less than that of cardinals, and is very largely merged in that of the more general conception of relation numbers.[4]

It seems perfectly obvious to me that this point of view is not correct. Ordinal numbers are more important and fundamental than cardinal numbers.

5 Concept of counting

The subject of counting is individual objects as a set or class – the number of apples in a bowl, eggs in a basket, children in a classroom. These are the cardinal numbers, as Frege calls them, e.g. the number of bricks and balls to play with. These numbers are drilled into children by parents and teachers.

The children are being prepared for doing business, since money has to be counted and wares too. The farmer counts the numbers of animals in his flocks and herds, using the cardinal numbers. Paul Benacerraf gives an interesting account of two kinds of counting, using the transitive and intransitive meanings of the verb 'to count'. Transitive counting is counting individual objects of a set – counting the marbles. A patient about to undergo an anaesthetic is also often asked to count, but just to count the numbers in a sequence, since in this case there is no reference to any specific objects to be counted, i.e. no set is involved – this is intransitive counting.

There are other uses of counting which have nothing to do with sets, e.g. counting time, the minutes, the hours, the days, etc. Heidegger refers to this use of counting towards the end of his *Being and Time*. But then we hardly need Heidegger to tell us about counting the time, it is part of everyone's knowledge and experience. Frege remarks at the end of his article on 'Numbers and Arithmetic' – written near the end of his life – that counting, which arose psychologically out of the demands of business, has 'led the learned astray'.

6 The commutative law

A fundamental axiom of axiomatic set theory is the commutative law of multiplication. The definition of 'commutative' in *The Concise Oxford Dictionary* is 'unchanged in result by the interchange of the order of quantities'. With equations, e.g. 4 x 3 = 3 x 4, the order of the numbers makes no difference. Likewise, in symbolic form, $AB = BA$. The two expressions are equal, they are identical. But there are systems of algebra in which $AB \neq BA$ – i.e. the equations are not equal, they are not identical. Here, the order of multiplication makes a difference. This type of multiplication is the foundation of the mathematical formalism used in quantum mechanics. As the commutative law of multiplication is an axiom of set theory, non-commutative multiplication of cardinal numbers – i.e. set numbers – is impossible.

7 The concept of value-ranges

Giving a simple example of this concept:

$$X^2 = 9$$

This is true for values of X of +3 and –3 and false for all other values of X.
In another example, where $X = 3$ and $Y = 4$:

$$XY = 12$$
$$YX = 12 \text{ also}$$

The multiplication in these two equations is commutative. For non-commutative multiplication:

$$XY \neq YX$$

This cannot be accounted for in the concept of value-ranges because the values of X or Y are the same; the only difference is in the order of the numbers.

8 Cardinal numbers have no direct reference to time

A set of four or ten individual objects have nothing to do with time except the psychological necessity of the time taken to count them – i.e. to arrive at a cardinal number, the total number in the group or set. If a farmer has 60 cows in a field, then to calculate their total would take about one minute at the average rate of counting of one per second. Frege in his *Grundlagen* makes very explicit reference to this problem:

> Time is only a psychological necessity for numbering, it has nothing to do with the concept of numbers.[5]

and later on the same page:

> Points of time, again, are separated by time intervals, long or short, equal or unequal. All these are relationships which have absolutely nothing to do with number as such.

Husserl in his *Philosophy of Arithmetic* (1891) expressed the same opinion: number has nothing to do with time – except the time taken to count a set of individual objects or numbers of a set. Both Frege and Husserl are using the concept of cardinal numbers only. But in physics – especially in astronomy – the numbering of time is essential. Even in everyday life time and numbers are very closely associated – the face of a clock has the hours and minutes numbered on it, a calendar has all the days of the month in numbers, while the dates of the years are important numbers for daily life, for history, for physics and for astronomy. Therefore numbers for time are obviously essential, and to say that numbers have nothing to do with time is not only incorrect but absolutely ridiculous.

9 Formal logic

The foundation of formal logic is axiomatic theory or proof theory. For proof theory you require true premises, i.e. axioms and valid arguments. Kant's analytical a priori judgements and synthetic a priori judgements are both true of necessity, i.e. they are axioms – their negation is non-existent. Frege's theory of truth-functions – that every declarative sentence or proposition has two values or references, the True and the False – does not apply to axioms, which have only one reference – the True. In dialectical logic every proposition without exception is true or false. Therefore there are no axioms: every proposition is in principle falsifiable, which is in accord with Popper's theory of falsifiability. All theories to be scientific must be falsifiable, which is not the case with axiomatic set theory. This principle should apply to mathematics as well as physical science. This is why non-commutative algebras can be accommodated in dialectical logic, whereas they are impossible in formal logic, with its foundation on axioms. With dialectical logic you always have two states of affairs – what is the case and what is not the case – which is the basis of a theory of meaning, not of proof theory.

10 Concept of meaning in mathematics

In technical mathematics, i.e. in the detailed work of a professional mathematician, proofs of various theories appear to be essential. But for the philosophy of mathematics attention must be given to the problem of meaning. One can ask the question: what is the meaning of 0 and 1? What is the meaning of negative numbers and imaginary numbers, incorporating $\sqrt{-1}$ and complex and hypercomplex numbers? The answer to such questions is not sufficiently clear in axiomatic set theory, where the emphasis is merely on proof, not on meaning. An extreme example of the neglect or complete disregard of meaning can be seen in the work on the foundations of mathematics by David Hilbert. Axiomatic theory is central to his philosophy of mathematics, and he is able to say that the point, the line and the plane can just as well be replaced by 'table, chair and mug'. This appears to be the consequence of his extreme formalism. It is obviously completely unacceptable, and it is no exaggeration to say it is nonsense.

11 The application of mathematics

Strictly speaking there is no such subject as physics: it can only be mathematical physics. All theories in physics must find a mathematical expression. Similarly there is no philosophy of physics: it must be the philosophy of mathematical physics. The problem now arises of how and why mathematics can be applied to the natural physical world, the world of empirical reality. It would seem that the formal logic of mathematics is unable to answer this question, being directly precluded from giving any answer.

This is clearly explained by Ayer in Chapter IV (concerning the a priori) of his book *Language, Truth and Logic*:

> Having thus shown that there is no inexplicable paradox involved in the view that the truths of logic and mathematics are all of them analytic, we may safely adopt it as the only satisfactory explanation of their a priori necessity. And in adopting

it we vindicate the empiricist claim that there can be no a priori knowledge of reality. For we show that the truths of pure reason, the propositions which we show to be valid independently of all experience, are so only in virtue of their lack of factual content. To say that a proposition is true a priori is to say that it is a tautology and tautologies, though they may serve to guide us in our empirical search for knowledge, do not in themselves contain any information about any matter of fact.[6]

Propositions which are true a priori are axioms – the fundamental starting point of formal logic. Therefore mathematics as formal logic cannot explain why mathematics is applicable to physics – the attempt to do so is completely excluded. The ultimate goal of explanation in physics is a unified theory – a theory of everything. The question then is: what would be the mathematical formulation or symbolism required for such a unified theory? The formal logic of axiomatic set theory is totally incapable of answering that question. The same situation also applies to every other existing philosophy of mathematics. This is a very unsatisfactory state of affairs. One might argue that an adequate philosophy of mathematics should indicate in some way the mathematics required for the unified theory of physics.

12 The branches of mathematics

The principal branches of mathematics are arithmetic, algebra and geometry. Husserl's work on the philosophy of mathematics, the *Philosophy of Arithmetic*, was published in 1891. Frege's works on the philosophy of mathematics are in English. *The Foundations of Arithmetic*, published in 1884, and the *Basic Laws of Arithmetic*, the first volume of which was published in 1893 and the second in 1903. All these works are on the philosophy of arithmetic only; there is no philosophy of algebra or geometry.

Michael Dummett in his book *Frege – Philosophy of Mathematics* (1991) quotes a long passage from Frege's *Foundations of Arithmetic*; the following is part of it:

> For conceptual thought we can always assume the opposite of this or that geometrical axiom, without involving ourselves in any self contradictions when we draw deductive consequences from assumptions conflicting with intuition such as these. This possibility shows that the axioms of geometry are independent of one another and of the fundamental laws of logic and are therefore synthetic. Can one say the same of the fundamental principles of number? Does not everything collapse in confusion when we try denying one of them? Would thought itself then be possible? Does not the ground of arithmetic lie deeper than that of all empirical knowledge even than that of Geometry? The truths of arithmetic govern the domain of what is countable. This is the most comprehensive of all; for it is not only what is actual, not only what is intuitable, that belongs to it, but everything thinkable. Should not the laws of number then stand in the most intimate connection with those of thought?[7]

Dummett comments that 'the axioms of geometry' meant for Frege the axioms of Euclidean geometry. When Frege refers to 'synthetic' he means Kant's synthetic a priori. By the 'science of numbers' Frege means the cardinal numbers of arithmetic, the domain of the countable, i.e. the numbers used for counting individual members or objects of a class or set. At the end of the quotation Dummett comments that the fact that the axioms of geometry (Euclidean geometry) can be denied without contradiction does not prove that they are synthetic; it depends on what is meant by synthetic. Frege uses the term to mean synthetic a priori. But this is not correct. Kant's synthetic a priori judgements are true necessarily, they are axioms. They cannot be contradicted. According to Frege and to everyone who uses axiomatic set theory the laws of arithmetic are analytical a priori. Arithmetic is simply a development of logic – formal logic – and every proposition of arithmetic is a law of logic. The conclusion therefore is that because the axioms of Euclidean geometry can be denied giving non-Euclidean geometry, geometry cannot be included in the philosophy of mathematics. This is of course why the works of Husserl and Frege on the philosophy of mathematics are restricted to the philosophy of arithmetic – in effect to axiomatic set theory using only cardinal numbers.

But this state of affairs is completely unacceptable. How can you have a philosophy of mathematics without geometry? All the concepts associated with geometry – whether space is Euclidean or non-Euclidean, flat or curved, the dimensions of space – are also not considered, yet space of two, three or n-dimensions is of special importance in mathematics and its application to the physical world. Also non-commutative algebra is impossible in formal logic because the commutative law is contradicted – equations are equal and not equal. The equations of motion are equal and in some systems not-equal.

David Bell's book on Husserl contains a comprehensive chapter on the latter's *Philosophy of Arithmetic* of 1891. At the end of the chapter is a section headed 'Grounds for Dissatisfaction'. Bell describes four of these objections to Husserl's whole theory. In the first he states:

An investigation of the logical symbolic and objective aspects of *arithmetical* knowledge, he realised, must remain unacceptably naive in the absence of an antecedent understanding of (say) the nature of logic, language, knowledge, meaning, existence, and truth *in general*, and in 1895 it was precisely this understanding that Husserl lacked.[8]

In the second ground for dissatisfaction Bell states:

In the first volume of the *Philosophy of Arithmetic*, that is, Husserl had proceeded on the assumption, inherited from his teacher Weierstrass, that 'pure arithmetic (or pure analysis) is a science based entirely and exclusively on the concept of cardinal numbers. It needs no other kind of presupposition . . .' But as Husserl's investigation into logical aspects of arithmetic progressed, it became clear, as he wrote to Stumpf, that the opinion by which he was guided in [Volume 1 of the *Philosophy of Arithmetic*], to the effect that the concept of cardinal number forms the foundation of general arithmetic, soon proved false . . . The fact is that 'general arithmetic' (including analysis, theory of functions etc.) finds *application* to the cardinals (in 'number theory'), as well as to the ordinals, to continuous quantities, and to n-fold extensions (time, space, colour, force continua etc.).[9]

In short cardinal numbers are inadequate for a satisfactory philosophy of mathematics. David Bell in his chapter on Husserl's philosophy of arithmetic does not mention the very significant fact that Husserl was most emphatic that number (cardinal number) had nothing to do with the concept of time. The only relation with time was the purely accidental and psychological one of the time taken to count the individualism in the set, group or collective. This is exactly the same as Frege's view on the relation between time and number. This omission on Bell's part could be related to his statement in the preface to his book that he would not include any references to Husserl's theory of time. This is regrettable as the problem of the concept of time is one of, if not the most, fundamental issues in the whole of philosophy and the natural world. To leave it out is like *Hamlet* without the Prince of Denmark.

This concludes my very brief account of 12 points on axiomatic set theory and its foundation on cardinal numbers. I propose to try another account of the philosophy of mathematics based on the real number system – measure numbers – exclusively using dialectical logic, which has no axioms. The concept of set, class or group will not be used. Formal logic, which has as its foundation axioms, proof and validity, will also not be used.

2 The concept of number

The fundamental concept of mathematics is that of number. We must ask the question: what is the meaning of number?

Frege mentions three fundamental principles in the introduction to his *Foundations of Arithmetic*. The second one is: never ask for the meaning of a word in isolation, but only in the context of a proposition. In the first part of his paper *On Meaning and Reference* he is considering the fact that different words or expressions can have the same reference. This is in effect a judgement – a proposition or declarative sentence of identity, that different words can have the same meaning.

But similarly the same word can have different meanings. The word then must be considered in isolation. Therefore Frege's context principle is incorrect from the point of view of linguistic analysis. The fact that the same word can have different meanings is not covered in either the first or the second part – on truth-functions – of his paper *On Meaning and Reference*. It is covered perfectly and explicitly in Wittgenstein's dictum: the meaning of a word is its use in the language. Therefore the same word can have different uses, meanings or applications. The word 'number' has two uses or meanings: cardinal number, and real number. There are thus two kinds of numbers. Michael Dummett gives a perfect quotation from Frege's *Grundgesetze:*

> Having remarked in section 157 of Volume II that 'we have interpreted real numbers as ratios of quantities', he goes on to say:
>
> > Since cardinal numbers (*Anzahlen*) are not Ratios we have to distinguish them from positive whole numbers. It is therefore not possible to extend the domain of cardinal numbers to that of the real numbers; they are completely disjoint

domains. The cardinal numbers answer the question, 'How many objects of a given kind are there?', whereas the real numbers can be regarded as measurement numbers, which state how large a quantity is as compared with a unit quantity.[1]

It would be difficult to find a better description of the difference between cardinal and real numbers. I like the use of the word 'domain': it even sounds beautiful in the English language. Roger Penrose in his book *The Emperor's New Mind* (1989) neatly summarises the meaning of real numbers, in a section called '"Reality" of real numbers':

Setting aside the notion of computability, real numbers are called 'Real' because they seem to provide the magnitudes needed for the measurement of distance, angle, time, energy, temperature or of the numerous other geometrical and physical quantities.[2]

The word 'distance' means of course length or extension. In that short single sentence the author uses three different words to describe real numbers: magnitude, measurement and quantity. To this list of examples of the real numbers mass could be added. The three most fundamental uses of the real numbers for measurement from a purely mathematical point of view are length – i.e. extension – time and angle. In George Temple's excellent book *100 Years of Mathematics*[3] he begins the first part with the title 'Number', with the initial chapters on real numbers. That is, right from the beginning the author starts with the real numbers.

Temple's chapter on mathematical logic is number 16, the second from last, which seems rather strange. For a philosopher of mathematics one might think it should be the first chapter, or at least nearer the beginning. He has an interesting comment on the place of logic in mathematics:

Mathematics has no monopoly of logical reasoning and the function of logic in mathematics is critical rather than constructive. Logical analysis is indispensable for an examination of the strength of a mathematical structure, but it is useless for its conception and design.

This is a rather different point of view from that of the formal logicians who wish to maintain that mathematics and logic are identical.

Frege in a letter to Russell gives a very explicit account of how he proposes to define the real numbers:

He mentions it explicitly in his letter to Russell of 21 May 1903 saying, 'As it seems to me you (i.e. Russell) need a double transition:

(1) from the cardinal numbers (*Anzahlen*) to the rational numbers, and (2) from the latter to the real numbers generally. I wish to go straight from the cardinal numbers to the real numbers as ratios of quantities'.[4]

31

This appears to contradict Frege's previous account of the difference between cardinal and real numbers already quoted above. There he said that it is not possible to extend the domain of cardinal numbers to that of the real numbers because they are completely disjoint domains. Frege is correct that the two number systems are completely disjoint or different domains, but he cannot free himself of the concept of cardinal numbers because it is based on his whole concept of class logic, i.e. formal logic.

As cardinal numbers and real numbers are completely distinct and have different uses, I propose to study the real numbers without any reference to or derivation from the cardinal numbers. Michael Dummett in the last two sentences of his book on Frege's philosophy of mathematics states:

> Above all, Frege provided the most plausible general answer yet proposed to the fundamental question, 'What is mathematics?' For all his mistakes and omissions, he was the greatest philosopher of mathematics yet to have written.

There is no doubt that Frege was a great logician and made fundamental contributions to the philosophy of mathematics, but we must look for someone else to guide us in the philosophy and meaning of mathematics and its fundamental concepts. Who is it to be? It is not Husserl, Frege, Cantor, Hilbert, Whitehead or Russell but Sir William Rowan Hamilton. He was without doubt the greatest mathematician of the nineteenth century. It is necessary to give his full names, at least at his first mention, as there is a well-known Scottish philosopher – a logician – of the same name: Sir William Hamilton (1788–1856). My Hamilton is of course well known to professional mathematicians but perhaps not so well known to philosophers of mathematics. The second edition of Hilbert's *Philosophy of Mathematics* edited by Benacerraf and Putnan in 1983 has a comprehensive list of articles on the subject. At the end of the book there is a very long bibliography of 30 pages but no reference to Hamilton, which I find very surprising.

Sir William Rowan Hamilton was born in Ireland in 1805. He had a brilliant career at Trinity College, Dublin, excelling in mathematics and languages. Hamilton had no problem combining these two quite different disciplines, and the footnotes in his papers and books are in Greek, Latin, French and German, etc. He was appointed Professor of Astronomy and Astronomer Royal for Ireland in 1827 at the age of 22, while still an undergraduate. He published very important papers *On a General Method in Dynamics* in 1834. The fundamental importance of his theories on dynamics was not fully realised until they were used by Schrödinger in 1926 in quantum mechanics. Hamilton's famous discovery of quaternions is exactly dated 16 October 1843. His *Lectures on Quaternions* was published in 1853 and the *Elements of Quaternions* the year after his death, in 1866.

Hamilton published a long paper in the *Transactions of the Royal Irish Academy* in 1837. This is more easily accessible in Volume 3 of the

Mathematical Papers of Sir William Rowan Hamilton published by the Cambridge University Press in 1967. The full title of this paper is: *Theory of Conjugate Functions or Algebraic Couples; with a Preliminary and Elementary Essay in Algebra as the Science of Pure Time.* His ideas on 'Algebra as the Science of Pure Time' are further developed at the beginning of the preface to his *Lectures on Quaternions* of 1853.

Hamilton's paper of 1837 is in fact in three parts:

1 Conjugate Functions or Algebraic Couples – 1833.
2 On Algebra as the Science of Pure Time – 1835.
3 General Introductory Remarks – to the final form of his paper of 1837.

In the latter part Hamilton describes how Newton's work in algebra was based on the notion of fluxions, which involves the notion of time. Napier in his invention of logarithms used the concept of continuous progression. Hamilton speaks expressly of fluxions, velocities and times, and observes that:

> Lagrange considered algebra to be the Science of Functions and it is not easy to conceive a clearer or just idea of a function in this science than by regarding its essence as consisting in *a law connecting change with change.* But where change and progression are, there is time. The notion of time is, therefore, inductively found to be connected with existing algebra.[5]

In this brief quotation you feel you are in a different world from that of the philosophy of arithmetic of Husserl and Frege, with their categorical assertion that time has nothing whatever to do with number and mathematics. Of course they are living in the world of set theory, their numbers are cardinal numbers – the number of beans in a can or sheep in a field; a group, a class or a set of individual beings or members. The only relation with time there is the length of time it takes to count the members of the set.

The last paragraph of Hamilton's general introductory remarks gives his views on the concept and use of time in mathematics and is worth quoting in full:

> That the mathematical science of time when sufficiently unfolded and distinguished on the one hand from all actual outward chronology (or collections of recorded events and phenomenal marks and measures), and on the other hand from all dynamical science (or reasonings and results from the notion of cause and effect), will ultimately be found to be co-extensive and identical with algebra, so far as algebra itself is a science; is a conclusion to which the author has been led by all his attempts, whether to analyse what is scientific in algebra or to construct a science of pure time. It is a joint result of the inductive and deductive processes, and the grounds on which it rests could not be stated in a few general remarks. The author hopes to explain them more fully in a future paper; meanwhile he refers to

the present one, as removing (in his opinion) the difficulties of the usual theory of negative and imaginary quantities, or rather substituting a new theory of contra-positives and couples, which he considers free from those old difficulties, and which is deduced from the intuition or original mental form of timing; the opposition of the (so called) negative and positives being referred by him; not to the opposition of the operations of increasing and diminishing a *magnitude,* but to the simpler and more extensive contrast between the relations of *before* and *after,* or between the directions of *forward* and *backward* being used to suggest a theory of conjugate functions which gives reality and meaning to conceptions that were before imaginary, impossible or contradictory, but mathematicians had derived them from that bounded notion of magnitude, instead of the original and comprehensive thought of ORDER IN PROGRESSION.[6]

It is worth noticing that Hamilton's emphasis is on the concept of the meaning of negative numbers and imaginary numbers using $\sqrt{-1}$. He is using the concept of order in progression, but that does not mean that the concept of magnitude, i.e. quantity or measure numbers, is excluded from mathematics: both of these concepts are required. The concept of order in progression is of the ordinal character of number, i.e. ordinal numbers not cardinal numbers, which have no ordinal character of number unless put there as a secondary and accidental factor in number:

> To count, to measure and to order were for Hamilton three very different, though connected acts of thought. These aspects of nature were already dealt with by three different branches of science – arithmetic, metrology and algebra. Hamilton thought that in arithmetic number is best as an answer to the question 'how many?' It constitutes a science of multitude found in the relations more and fewer, or ultimately of the many and the one. Metrology is more concerned with measurement and magnitude, and so is essentially different from arithmetic. In algebra, Hamilton considered the role of number to be radically different again. Here he thought it really answers the question, 'How placed in succession?' If so, it inevitably suggests comparison with temporal order – the everyday experience of time, where we perceive events succeed each other regularly.[7]

The trio of concepts – counting, measuring or ordering – are not necessarily separate: in fact they are often combined. In any measure the counting applies to it both for time and extension; likewise the numbers used in measures are in order, they are ordinal numbers.

3 Number systems

I propose to examine the various number systems in the following order:

1 Real numbers
2 Complex numbers
3 Quaternions
4 Hypercomplex numbers

Real numbers

The real numbers have three different meanings:

1 Measure numbers
2 Ratio of qualities
3 Scalar numbers

We must answer the question: what do the real numbers measure? The two most fundamental measures are space – i.e. extension, or length – and time. The measurement of angle is also fundamental for mathematics. In physics and mathematical physics mass, temperature and speed are important measure numbers.

In the measurement of space – i.e. extension – we are concerned with the space of the universe, the cosmos as a whole, as one unity, one reality. We are not concerned with the measure – extension – of particular individual objects, e.g. the extension or length of a room or garden, the length of a table, the diameter of a tennis ball. In the same way we are concerned with time in the universe as a whole – again the cosmos, which is existing in time. Time can be predicted of the whole universe, since modern cosmology can give a number for the age of the universe or cosmos: it is estimated to be 15,000,000,000 years old. Again we are not concerned with the time or age of individual objects, the life span of human beings or animals, the age of a house, or the duration of a football match. We are only concerned with time in the universe, which conceptually can be thought of as extending to infinity in both directions.

It may seem odd to include time in a work on mathematics and the philosophy of mathematics. In George Temple's book *100 Years of Mathematics,* there is a large section – Part II – headed 'Space', with several chapters, but there is no chapter on time. The subject of dynamics, on the other hand, is the study of motion in time. As already mentioned, Hamilton considered that the essence of a function consists of a law connecting change with change – and where there is change there is time. We can think of the universe as one reality, one thing existing in space and time, and not as individual objects.

In Russell's introduction to Wittgenstein's *Tractatus* (1961) he makes the criticism that:

> there is no way whatever according to him by which we describe the totality of things that can be named, in other words the totality of what there is in the world. In order to be able to do this we should have to know some property which must belong to every thing by a logical necessity.

Russell mentions the totality of things – this is his logical atomism. But there is only one thing, the real universe. Later he comments on what he calls Wittgenstein's fundamental thesis, that it is impossible to say anything about the world as a whole. This is of course completely incorrect. The universe as a whole exists in space – which is its extension – and exists in time – whether time had a beginning or whether the universe exists from all eternity. They are both predicates of the whole universe – the cosmos.

The real numbers as measure numbers can be called scalar numbers. This term was first used by Hamilton. The numbers are on a scale – a line extending from – infinity to + infinity.

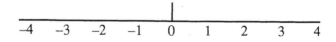

It is clearly evident that measure numbers, or scalar numbers, are ordinal numbers by their very nature or essence. In this they are completely different from cardinal numbers, which, as set numbers, have no ordinal character. The ordinal numbers have no relationship to the concept of a set or group. You could think of points on a line as a set, but that seems completely artificial and unnecessary.

All measure numbers are ordinal numbers, not just the numbers representing the progression of time – as Hamilton would say, there is order in progression. The operation of counting applies to measure numbers. It is perhaps most obvious with the counting of time. It is also easy to see with the counting of length, e.g. of a piece of cloth. With a one-metre measure you can count the numbers of metres in the dimensions of a room.

There is no problem with the meaning of 0: it is the point of origin of a scale, as is obvious with measures of length and weight. The number 0 is at the beginning of the scale, it has nothing to do with a set or class which has no members. In the measuring of temperature 0 is the freezing point of water in the Celsius scale. Temperature has an absolute scale in degrees Kelvin; $-273°C$ is absolute zero. A temperature of $-10°K$ is non-existent. Different types of measures can have different scales – Celsius and Fahrenheit for temperature, metres and yards for length, and pounds and kilograms for mass. This leads to the problem of matching the two scales and their standards. (The problem of the scales of time will be considered later.) This is all related to the meaning of 1 as the basic unit of measurement. It has nothing to do with only one member of a class or set.

The multiplication of real numbers is commutative; the order of multiplication does not affect the result:

$$4 \times 3 = 3 \times 4$$

If you have three rods each four metres long laid in a line it makes 12 metres. Four rods each three metres long and laid in a line also makes 12 metres.

On the scale of real numbers a place can always be found for the rational numbers ½ , ¼, etc. on the line of the sequence of numbers. The same applies to irrational numbers, e.g. $\sqrt{2}$. This means that the scale of real numbers is infinitely divisible. There are infinite numbers of points between any integer, e.g. between 1 and 2 and 2 and 3.

Summary of real numbers

1 Measure numbers measure length in space, time, angles, mass, temperature and speed. They are all scalar numbers.
2 Scalar numbers lie on a scale from minus infinity to plus infinity. They are in one dimension.
3 Numbers are ordinal by their very nature.
4 0 is the point of origin of a scale.
5 1 is the unit of measurement.
6 Numbers can be counted.

7 Multiplication is commutative.

8 Numbers are infinitely divisible.

9 Numbers are infinitely extended, i.e. transfinite ordinal numbers.

10 They are single numbers.

Complex numbers

Understanding the meaning of complex numbers is a special problem for philosophers who have no special technical knowledge of mathematics. These numbers are very familiar and simple for professional mathematicians, but their original discovery and explanation was far from simple. Complex numbers involve an investigation into the meaning of imaginary numbers, e.g. $\sqrt{-1}$ and negative numbers, e.g. -1. This is best illustrated by means of a few simple equations:

$$X^2 + 1 = 0$$
$$X^2 = -1$$
$$X = \sqrt{-1}$$

The problem here is what is the meaning of $\sqrt{-1}$? It is an imaginary number: it appears to mean nothing in reality. The first explanation of the problem was a geometrical one. To demonstrate this, we can use the Argand plane with Cartesian coordinates, the horizontal axis being the real axis and the vertical axis the imaginary axis:

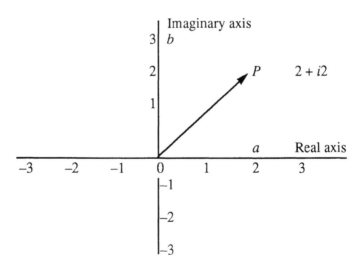

The symbol $i = \sqrt{-1}$

38

The point P on the plane is $2 + i2$ or in more general symbolic form $a + ib$. This geometrical explanation of imaginary numbers was well known to Hamilton, but he was not satisfied with this explanation and wanted an explanation less dependent on geometry. This was achieved in his paper of 1833 on *Conjugate Functions or Algebraic Couples*. In this he showed that complex numbers can be expressed as ordered pairs of real numbers which obey all the rules or operations of addition, division and multiplication.

The following diagram is useful in this explanation:

		Imaginary axis	
+1		0.1	
−1.0		1.0	Real axis
	−1 0 +1		
		0.−1	
−1			

Therefore:

$$1 = 1.0$$
$$\sqrt{-1} = 0.1$$
$$-1 = -1.0$$
$$-\sqrt{-1} = 0.-1$$

In general symbolism the ordered pairs (or couples as Hamilton called them) are expressed a, b or a_1, a_2 and $ab = a + ib$, i.e. a complex number. The $\sqrt{-1}$ or i cannot be given a meaning with a single number: it must be an ordered pair or couple, i.e. two numbers are required. This seems very elementary and simple for professional mathematicians, but Hamilton was the first to give $\sqrt{-1}$ and complex numbers that explanation. He arrived at this explanation through the concept of time with a motion forward and backward in time. He developed this further in his paper *On Algebra as the Science of Pure Time* of 1835. (This will be described later.) With Hamilton's description of complex numbers as ordered pairs of real numbers, the imaginary number $\sqrt{-1}$ has disappeared – there is nothing imaginary in the concept of the ordered pairs, or couples, of real numbers.

In the first diagram of the Argand plane the point P is the order pair $a.b$ or in the diagram $a + ib$. But it can also be represented as the line from the origin 0 to the point P. This is a line or step from 0 to P, a directed line with a certain length. You can in your imagination carry the point 0 along the line to P. Hamilton was the first to call this directed line a vector, from the Latin *vehere*, to carry. This he describes in his first *Lecture on Quaternions*.

We now have a completely new concept of number: a directed line in space of two dimensions – i.e. a real number with a direction, a vector. The concept of a vector is of supreme importance in mathematics, in physics and, I believe, in the philosophy of mathematics.

But if you think of complex numbers only as ordered pairs of real numbers, the concept of a directed number is completely absent, and you miss the directed character of a vector.

Using a vector we can give clear meaning to the numbers –1 and √–1. In the following diagram the Cartesian coordinates are in a circle:

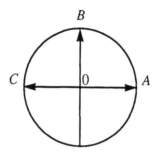

Multiplying the vector 0A by –1 rotates it through 180°, i.e. π radians to point C: it is now the vector 0C, a negative number. Therefore –1 is an operator which operates on a single vector, rotating it by convention in a leftward or anticlockwise direction by 180° – two right angles – to generate a negative number. Then √–1 is an operator which operates on the same single vector 0A, rotating it through one right angle – 90° – or π/2 radians to B. Repeating the operation the vector 0B is rotated through another right angle – 90° – to 0C, which is the negative of 0A.

That is, √–1 x √–1 = –1, which gives clear meaning to the imaginary number √–1. It is concerned with the rotation of vectors.

A complex number can thus have three different meanings:

1 An ordered pair of real numbers a, b.
2 The sum of a real and imaginary number $a + ib$.
3 A vector – a directed magnitude, a real number with direction in two dimensions.

From a philosophical point of view the concept of a complex number as a vector is of more interest and importance, which will be more evident later.

The motion of translation can be in any number of different directions – north, south, east and west and to all points of the circle – in the limit: therefore motion can be in an infinite number of directions. But in rotation or intrinsic spin there are only two possible directions – left-handed or anticlockwise, and right-handed or clockwise.

Once you have the concept of a vector – i.e. a directed line in space of two dimensions – operations on it can be considered. The vector can increase in length, i.e. undergo a change of length. Hamilton called this by the name 'tensor'. This word is derived from the Latin *tendere*, to stretch – i.e. to increase in length. It is like a piece of elastic which by stretching increases in length. That is the correct etymological use of the word 'tensor'. The word 'tensor' as it appears in the tensor calculus used in general relativity is obviously completely different: here it is a generalised vector, and has no relation to the correct meaning of the word.

Hamilton then uses the word 'versor' for the turning or rotating of a vector, described earlier – again the correct use of the language, which is only what you expect from Hamilton.

The multiplication of vectors thus has two different meanings. The first is the increase of the length of the vector – the tensor. This multiplication is commutative, just as it is for real numbers. The second type of multiplication is round a point, or rotation. The rotation to the right and to the left is equal when you have a change of angle, the versor. This multiplication is also commutative.

Frege in his *Foundations of Arithmetic* (1884) has no adequate account of complex numbers. At the beginning of section 92 – that is, almost at the end of the book – he says, 'up to now we have restricted our treatment to the natural numbers', i.e. the cardinal numbers. In Section 100 he mentions the moon multiplied by itself as -1. This gives us a square root of -1 in the shape of the moon! This is complete nonsense. Later he says let us choose as our square root of -1 the time interval of 1 second symbolised by i. Thus $3i$ will mean the time interval of 3 seconds. This is again nonsense.

Russell in his *Introduction to Mathematical Philosophy* (1919) describes a complex number as simply an ordered couple of real numbers. But there is no mention that it is a vector – a directed magnitude in two dimensions. The concept of rotation of a cardinal number is totally impossible; the possibility is non-existent. The same applies to the real numbers, i.e. scalars, which are single numbers. Only vectors can rotate because they are real numbers which have direction. Vector numbers are absolutely essential in their application to physics to describe measures which have direction. The physical quantities which have direction are acceleration force, velocity and momentum, both linear momentum and angular momentum. Vectors are therefore measure numbers, of magnitude and direction.

Summary of complex numbers

1 They can be ordered pairs (couples) of real numbers in two dimensions.
2 They can be vectors – real numbers with direction in two dimensions.
3 They can give meaning given to negative numbers and $\sqrt{-1}$.

4   Multiplication of vectors is of two types:

 a)   change of magnitude or length of vector
 b)   rotation around a point.

5   This multiplication is commutative.
6   They are measure numbers, they measure velocity, acceleration force and momentum – all of which have magnitude and direction.

Quaternions

Understanding quaternions for a philosopher who has no special knowledge of mathematics is quite a problem. Even some professional mathematicians have some difficulty in fully understanding them and their applications and meaning. They were of course Hamilton's famous discovery. The solution of the difficulties he faced came to him in a flash of inspiration on 16 October 1843.

Complex numbers are ordered pairs – or couples, as Hamilton called them – of real numbers. They are also vectors in space of two dimensions. It seemed to Hamilton an obvious step to develop the number system to apply to the three dimensions of ordinary space using triplets instead of couples. He tried to solve the problem for many years. There is the well-known story about his coming down to breakfast every morning. His young sons would ask him: 'Papa, can you multiply triplets?' He always answered: 'No, I can add and subtract them, but I cannot multiply them.' Then finally the correct answer came to him. Two special steps were required in the correct solution of his problem. The first was that a set of four numbers was required, not three, and the commutative law of multiplication had to be abandoned. The multiplication of real numbers and complex numbers is commutative, so to abandon this law was a great break with mathematical tradition. Hamilton came to see that geometrical operations in three-dimensional space required for their description not triplets but quadruplets – i.e. a set of four numbers; if we consider, for example, the operation which when performed on one vector a converts it into another vector, we see that in order to specify this operation we need to know the ratio of the length of a, and b the angle between them, and the node and inclination of the plane in which they lie – that is, four numbers altogether. Hamilton called the set of four numbers a quaternion. The word is used for the squad of four soldiers guarding St Peter as recorded in the Authorised Version of the New Testament, Acts 12:4.

The non-commutative law is expressed in Hamilton's symbolism:

$$ji = -ji$$

E.T. Whittaker comments on this most important discovery in an article

42

'The Sequence of Ideas in the Discovery of Quaternions', originally written in 1943 to celebrate the centenary of their discovery:

> This was the supreme moment in the history of mathematical symbolism. It began the creative process which yielded not only quaternions, but all the other systems which broke from the old rules – Cayley and Sylvester's matrices, Boole's symbolic logic, Grassmann's *Ausdehnungslehre*, Gibbs' dyadics, and the Heisenberg–Dirac algebra of quantum mechanics.[1]

To explain the symbolism Hamilton used it is useful to go back to the diagram used to explain complex numbers:

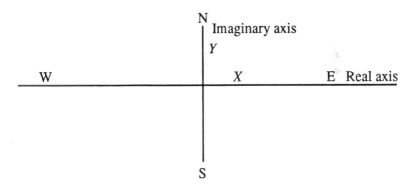

There is one imaginary axis – north–south – and one real axis – east–west. In quaternions all three axes of space are imaginary:

1 North–south – $+j$ and minus j.
2 East–west – $+i$ and minus i.
3 Up and down – $+k$ and minus k, i.e. above the level of the paper and below the level of the paper.

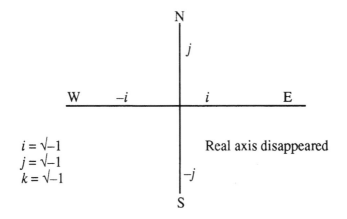

In this symbolism all three axes in space are imaginary – the real axis which was in the complex number diagram has disappeared. The fourth number of the quaternion is a real number, a scalar number.

The formula for a quaternion is:

$$q = s + ia + jb + kc$$

If any two of a, b, c are zero you have a complex number:
If $b + c$ are zero
$\quad s + ia$ is a complex number.
If a, b and c are zero
$\quad s$ is a real number or scalar number.

Therefore quaternions include the real and complex numbers as special cases. They are an extension of complex numbers from two to three dimensions. The fundamental formula of quaternions is:

$$i^2 = j^2 = k^2 = ijk = -1$$

This is obvious since i, j and k are each $= \sqrt{-1}$. The symbolism for non-commutative multiplication is expressed as follows:

1 $\quad ij = -ji = k$
2 $\quad jk = -kj = i$
3 $\quad ki = -ik = j$

Using the first line only as an example:

$ij = +k; (-ji = k) \times -1$ gives $ji = -k$
$ji = -k$

If $ij = -ji$
then $ij + ji = +k - k = 0$

The non-commutative multiplication of the first line $ij = -ij$ is clearly explained in words by Sean O'Donnell in his book *William Rowan Hamilton*:

It (the famous commutative law) was one of those things apparently so natural that everybody before Hamilton had assumed that it must always be true. Basically, the commutative law merely formalised the seemingly obvious truth that 3 x 2 must always equal 2 x 3. This means that the *order* of multiplication can be changed or commuted without affecting the result. Whether you start with a 2 or a 3 had always seemed immaterial, a principle built into the very foundation of algebra as the commutative law.

In quaternions, however, it now emerges that the order of multiplication matters very much indeed. Remembering that multiplication is equivalent to rotation in these matters one can again appreciate this issue in solution of the Rubik cube puzzle. There the challenge is to get the order or sequence of rotation (multiplication) absolutely right.

A century and a half ago Hamilton was the first to appreciate this issue mathematically. Suppose for example that you rotate the northward line about the eastward line as previously. Then the appropriate algebraic statement is:

$ij = k$ (upwards)

If, however, you now alter the sequence in the first part of this equation, a very different result is obtained. Since j is written first this time, it now becomes the operator round which i is rotated. In other words, the eastward line i, is turned about northward one j. And since such rotation is always leftward in our convention, the end position of the former is obviously downward or denoted by $-k$. Expressed algebraically we then have:

$ji = -k$ (downwards)

A result obviously different from the previous one.[2]

The operation involves the rotation of vectors in three dimensions. The rotations are multiplications. The operation ij results in the vector ending in the direction upwards, i.e. $+k$. The operation ji results in the same vector ending in the direction downwards, i.e. $-k$.

The order of the multiplication affects the result. At the end of the first operation the vector is pointing upwards, at the end of the second the same vector is pointing downwards – they are in opposite directions.

Mary Hesse in her book *Science and the Human Imagination* (1954) gives a neat and simple example of the difference the order of an operation can make. If you have a dinner before crossing the Channel in a gale you are likely to feel ill. If you have the dinner after the rough crossing you will not be ill. The order of the operation makes a difference. But she did not complete the story. You can ask what the circumstance would be if taking the meal before or after the crossing made no difference? The answer of course is if there was no wind and the crossing was very smooth. There are two states of affairs corresponding to the order in which operations are carried out – in symbolic form $AB = BA$ and $AB \neq BA$.

In the second equation the multiplication is non-commutative. The word as used here is an adjective. In its verbal form we would say that the equation commutes or does not commute. The noun form is commutativity, but this sounds awkward, and a better word might be commutability. In axiomatic set theory the commutative law for cardinal numbers is an axiom:

$AB = BA$

In other words, the equation commutes. The concept of the equation being not equal is a logical impossibility. This is pointed out by Susan Stebbing:

> There are non commutative algebras for which the second principle [principle of commutation *AB=BA*] does not hold. So long as the basis of arithmetic, and therefore of algebra, is based upon our intuitions with regard to *counting*, non commutative algebras will seem absurd, just as, so long as geometrical axioms are based upon our intuitions of space, non Euclidean geometrics will seem absurd. These formal principles stand to algebra as Euclidean axioms to geometry.[3]

By 'counting' of course, she means counting individual objects or members of a set, i.e. cardinal numbers. By 'formal principles' she means axioms, i.e. propositions which are true of necessity, whose negation is logically impossible.

Frege's principle of value-ranges is of no help with non-commutative multiplication, e.g. $x^2 = 9$. This is true for values of x of +3 and −3 and false for all other values of x.

But for $AB = BA$ and $AB \neq BA$ the values of A and B in both commutative and non-commutative multiplication are the same in each case. The only difference is in the order of the symbols representing numbers. The equations commute and do not commute, i.e. we have two states of affairs which are contradictory, divided by a negation. This is impossible in logic based on axioms, i.e. formal logic. With dialectical logic both the states of affairs can exist – what is the case and what is not the case. With $AB = BA$ you have an equation, i.e. an identity, whereas with $AB \neq BA$ the equation is not equal, you have a difference. We must now list all the conditions for the non-commutability of multiplication in quaternions:

1   Numbers must be vectors, i.e. have direction in space.
2   Multiplication in quaternions involves rotation.
3   The dimensions of space in which quaternions operate are three.

As a consequence of these three conditions the order of multiplication makes a difference. Non-commutative multiplication with the cardinal numbers of set theory is impossible. The first condition is absent – cardinal numbers have no direction. The second condition is also absent – the concept of cardinal numbers rotating is also impossible.

The third condition is again absent – cardinal numbers have no relationship to the three dimensions of space. The same applies to the real numbers. They have no directed character, they cannot be rotated and they have no relation to the three dimensions of space. They are scalar numbers in one dimension. Complex numbers also do not fulfil the conditions for non-commutative multiplication as they are vectors in two dimensions only. It is worth commenting at this point on a text of the late Alfred Ayer:

For example, in physics it is not always safe to apply the commutative law that axb is equivalent to bxa. If the quantities are vectors, it makes a difference in which order they are taken.[4]

This is of course a very serious error. Vectors are complex numbers in two dimensions and their multiplication is commutative, the same as for real numbers. It is only when the vectors are in three dimensions that their multiplication is non-commutative. Did Ayer ever hear of Sir William Rowan Hamilton and his quaternions, the first example and discovery of non-commutative algebra? Ayer's contribution to the philosophy of mathematics is contained in Chapter IV of his *Language, Truth and Logic* (1946). This is considered important enough to be included in the comprehensive collection of essays on Hilbert's *Philosophy of Mathematics* (1983), edited by Benacerraf and Putnan. But there is no mention of non-commutative algebra in that account of the philosophy of mathematics.

We now reconsider the fundamental equation of quaternions which Hamilton discovered in a flash of inspiration on 16 October 1843:

$$i^2 = j^2 = k^2 = ijk = -1$$

Since i, j and k are each equal to $\sqrt{-1}$, it is clear that their squares are each equal to -1.

But how does $ijk = -1$? If the symbols are expressed separately, then each is equal to $\sqrt{-1} \times \sqrt{1} \times \sqrt{-1} = -\sqrt{-1}$, and this is not the correct result. The expression ijk can be given three different forms:

1 $i \times jk$
2 $j \times ki$
3 $k \times ij$

Thus, jk, ki, ij are each operations of multiplication. The equations for multiplication are:

1 $jk = -kj = i$
2 $ki = -ik = j$
3 $ij = -ji = k$

By substituting i for jk, j for ki, and k for ij, the expression ijk gives:

1 $i \times i = -1$
2 $j \times j = -1$
3 $k \times k = -1$

which is what is required to show:

$$ijk = -1$$

Mathematicians whose works I have read state that quaternions represent space of four dimensions. This is incorrect. Three of the numbers of the set of four used in quaternions represent space of three dimensions: east–west, north–south and up and down, i.e. vectors in three directions of space. The problem then is what does the fourth number – a real number – represent? It has been suggested that the fourth number represents time. Hamilton wrote a sonnet on quaternions, from which the following two lines come: 'and how the one of time, of space the three,/ Might in the chain of symbol girdled be'.

Hamilton makes other reference to time in some letters about quaternions. Cornelius Lanczos commented on this particular problem:

> The renowned physicist, Cornelius Lanczos, has put this aspect unequivocally. 'It is astonishing to see how the quaternions of Hamilton foreshadowed our four dimensional world, in which space and time are united into a single entity, the 'space time' world of Einstein's Relativity. Today we are inclined to call d the 'time part' and ai + bj + ck the 'space part' of the quaternion q.' Lanczos goes further in suggesting that quaternions provide the exact tool nowadays for all problems involving some kind of rotation in the four dimensional world.[5]

Lanczos also is referring to the four-dimensional world. But the world has three and only three dimensions of space – the fourth number must refer to something else, and that could be time, which has no relationship to space. Hamilton in his *Elements of Quaternions* described hundreds of applications of his quaternions to physics. But there is one particular area in which their application is most fitting and that is for the study of the dynamics of tops and gyroscopes – i.e. spin. Angular momentum has two categories: orbital angular momentum, and intrinsic spin angular momentum. Orbital angular momentum can be described by complex numbers, i.e. vectors in two dimensions only. But intrinsic spin angular momentum requires not two but three dimensions of space. The intrinsic spin of a body can be in the three dimensions of space. The axis of spin can be:

1 East–west.
2 North–south.
3 Up and down – i.e. along a vertical axis.

This can be demonstrated so simply that any child can see it. A knitting needle can be put through an apple. The direction of the needle is the axis of spin for the apple. It is clearly evident that the needle – the axis of spin – can be pointing in the three directions of space: east–west, north–south, and with the needle in the vertical position – up and down. We can now jump from the apple with the needle through the middle to the spin of electrons in quantum mechanics.

E.T. Whittaker has commented on this application:

> Thus the 'spin matrices' introduced by Pauli in 1927, on which the quantum mechanical theory of rotations and angular momenta depend, are simply Hamilton's three quaternions units i. j. k. Professor Conway has shown in an interesting paper that quaternion methods may be used with advantage in the discussion of Dirac's equation for the spinning electron: and the formalism of 1843 may even yet prove to be the most natural expression of the new physics.[6]

But the description of spin with three symbols for the three axes of spin is not complete. You need to know the rate of spin. This of course includes time – the number of revolutions per minute, for example – and also the direction of the spin – i.e. right-handed or left-handed. This could be the fourth unit of quaternions – a real number, a scalar number. Hamilton considered a quaternion to be a scalar plus a vector. With this concept in mind he had at one time thought of calling it a grammarithm. (*Gramma* is the Greek word for line, and *arithmos* is number – meaning a line and a number, i.e. a vector plus a scalar.) Quaternions would thus seem to be the perfect and complete number system. It is a perfect union of algebra and geometry, which combines the complex numbers with the three dimensions of space within the real numbers.

Summary of quaternions

1 They involve an extension of the number system to the three dimensions of space with one real number – which could be time.

2 In quaternions the multiplication is non-commutative. This is the most important aspect of quaternions for logic and the philosophy of mathematics. The concept of non-commutative multiplication is impossible in axiomatic set theory – i.e. for cardinal numbers. Their equations can be equal and not equal, i.e. they commute and do not commute. This concept is only possible with the use of dialectical logic, where the two states of affairs are possible – what is the case and what is not the case.

3 Quaternions have direct application to intrinsic angular momentum, or spin. They are measure numbers for spin.

Hypercomplex numbers

Complex numbers are vectors in two dimensions, quaternions are vectors in three dimensions. A natural extension to our number systems is to consider vectors in dimensions greater than three, i.e. up to n-dimensions – in other words, hypercomplex numbers. The vectors can be represented as sets of numbers, e.g. a_1, a_2; this can be extended, e.g. a_1, a_2, a_3, a_4, a_n. Quaternions are often called hypercomplex numbers. They are also said to represent four-dimensional space, which is not correct. Quaternions in fact symbolise the three dimensions of the space of the natural or real world, while their fourth number could symbolise time. The term hypercomplex number should therefore be reserved for numbers symbolising dimensions of space greater than three, or up to n-dimensions, whereas the term quaternions should be kept as a separate and unique category. The extension of the number concept to n-dimensions was carried out by Grassmann (1844) in his work *Ausdehnungslehre*. This is a theory of extension or 'extended magnitudes', which can be interpreted as a generalised vector analysis for space of n-dimensions. The work is so generalised that it includes quaternions as a special case. This extension of the number concept was also made by Arthur Cayley (1821–1895) with his theory of matrices. Quaternions can also be represented in matrix form. The special feature of matrices is that their multiplication is non-commutative – this is their special interest for logic and the philosophy of mathematics and for physics. This was the non-commutative algebra used by Heisenberg, Born and Jordan in 1925 in their theory of matrix mechanics as applied to quantum mechanics:

> We now make the further assumption that *the linear operators correspond to the dynamical variables at that time*. By dynamical variables are meant quantities such as the co-ordinates and the components of velocity, momentum and angular momentum of particles, and functions of these quantities – in fact the variables in terms of which classical mechanics is built up. The new assumption requires that these quantities shall occur also in quantum mechanics, but with the striking difference that they are now subject to an algebra in which the commutative axiom of multiplication does not hold.
> This different algebra for the dynamical variables is one of the most important ways in which quantum mechanics differs from classical mechanics.[7]

This radical difference between classical mechanics and gravitation and quantum mechanics is of the most fundamental importance for logic and the philosophy of mathematics and physics. Dirac talks of the 'commutative axiom of multiplication not holding'. For axiomatic set theory the commutative axiom does hold, meaning that its negation is impossible – this is because an axiom is a proposition which is true of necessity.

The fundamental formula of quantum mechanics is:

$$pq = qp = ih/2\pi$$

Here q is the coordinate specifying the position of a particle, e.g. an electron, and p is the momentum of the particle. In classical mechanics $pq = qp$ or $pq - qp = 0$. In classical mechanics the equations of motion are equal, they commute. Therefore the order of multiplication of p and q makes no difference. In quantum mechanics the order of multiplication does make a difference: the equations of motion are not equal, they do not commute. In the standard Copenhagen interpretation the intervention of measuring instruments prevents one from obtaining exact values of the position and momentum of a particle simultaneously because the particles are so minute. This results in Heisenberg's Uncertainty Principle, where position and momentum cannot both be known with a greater degree of accuracy than is specified by a limit expressed in terms of Planck's constant. But when the particle or object to be measured is very massive – such as a planet or the moon – the disturbance is negligible and $h/2\pi$ is zero. This is why the equations of motion commute in classical mechanics but do not commute in quantum mechanics. Therefore the unification of classical mechanics and quantum mechanics appears to be logically impossible: the two theories are contradictory.

We must now consider what is the meaning of the non-commutative algebra of matrices used in quantum mechanics and how and why it is different from the non-commutative character of Hamilton's quaternions. A suggested answer is given by E.T. Whittaker in his address as President of the Royal Society of Edinburgh on 25 October 1943. The title of the address was 'The New Algebras and Their Significance for Physics and Philosophy'. The substance of this address is also contained in Section 57 of his published *Tarner Lectures*. By coincidence the very month and year of his address are the centenary of the discovery of quaternions by Hamilton in 1843. Whittaker refers to this at the beginning of his address and describes Hamilton's discovery of non-commutative algebra. Whittaker had a profound knowledge of Hamilton's work, and had the same appointment as Hamilton from 1906 to 1912 when he was Professor of Astronomy at Trinity College, Dublin and Astronomer Royal for Ireland. He had special knowledge of Hamilton's theory of dynamics and his quaternions. In his 1943 address he summarised in one sentence the new algebras and their significance, i.e. their meaning for physics and philosophy. In the philosophy of mathematics the fundamental objective is meaning not proof. 'Non-commutative algebra is, in fact, the symbolism appropriate to things that cannot be measured exactly.'[8] 'Things that are not measured exactly' – that is a move away from precision in quantum mechanics. This is the concept of imprecision – the mathematical representation of Heisenberg's Uncertainty Principle. In quantum mechanics the equations of motion do not commute – that is imprecision. In classical mechanics the equations of motion do commute – that is precision. In the non-commutative multiplication of quaternions, the element of imprecision is totally absent. Why is that different from the non-commutative multiplication of the matrices used in quantum theory? As already described, one of the conditions for non-commutative multiplication was the number of dimensions of space involved. In quaternions there are the three dimensions of space, whereas in matrix algebra there are n-dimensions – i.e. Hilbert's space – a theory of vectors in a space of infinite dimensions. That is the reason for the difference between quaternions and matrix algebra.

51

Complex numbers are in two dimensions of space and their multiplication is commutative. We now ask the question is it possible to make the multiplication of complex numbers (vectors) non-commutative? I believe the answer is yes, it is possible. In Hamilton's definition of vectors the versor is the change of angle in the rotation of the vector and the tensor is the stretching or the change of length of the vector. If there is continuous change of angle only the versor, the point of the vector, can generate a circle – left rotation and right rotation are equal, i.e. commutative multiplication:

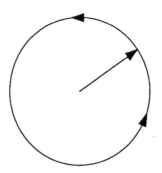

But if there is a change of length, or tensor, as well as a change of angle, or versor, a spiral is generated. Then left-hand rotation is different from right-hand rotation; the multiplication here is non-commutative – the order of the multiplication makes a difference:

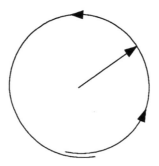

If a body is moving in a closed circle the equation of motion is commutative, the equation commutes. If the body is moving in a spiral, the equation of motion is non-commutative, the equation does not commute or the equation is anticommuting. By extending the concept of angle, or versor, of a vector in the third dimension of space a helix can be generated, i.e. a spiral in three dimensions and in two directions, left-handed or right-handed.

Further consideration must be given to the possible physical meaning of quaternion multiplication with special reference to spin or intrinsic angular momentum. In the following example, the three quaternion units i, j, k represent the three axes of spin of a body such as a top or gyroscope:

$$ij = + k$$

If the vector is upwards, i.e. the axis of spin is upwards and the direction of spin is, say, left-handed or anticlockwise:

$$ji = -k$$

If the vector is changed to downwards, i.e. the axis of spin is downwards, the direction of spin will now change to right-handed or clockwise. Therefore ij represents left-handed spin and ji right-handed spin. With spin there are two and only two possible directions. It is clear there is no element of imprecision in this operation. The non-commutative multiplication then represents a change in the direction of spin from left to right or right to left, as the case may be.

The following is a summary in tabular form of the different number systems and their commutability and the corresponding area of measurement. The numbers are always vectors, i.e. real numbers which have direction in space. The difference between them is due to the number of dimensions in each case. In commutative multiplication the order of multiplication makes

Dimension	Number systems	Commutability	Measure numbers
1	Real numbers	Commutative	Scalar Length, time, mass, temperature, angle
2	Complex numbers		
	a) change of angle only	a) commutative	a) orbital angular momentum
	b) change of angle and change of length	b) non-commutative	b) orbital angular momentum in spiral
3	Quaternions	Non-commutative	Intrinsic angular momentum or spin
n	Hypercomplex numbers, matrices	Non-commutative	Probability of imprecision

no difference. In non-commutative multiplication the order does make a difference – this is the essence of the concept of commutability.

The very word 'real' means the applicability of the numbers to the real natural world. Frege has made an explicit reference to this in his criticism of the formalist approach to the philosophy of mathematics in Volume II, Section 91 of his *Grundgesetze*: 'It is applicability alone that raises arithmetic from the rank of a game to that of a science, applicability therefore belongs to it of necessity.'[9]

This concept of applicability involves not only arithmetic, but all branches of mathematics. But Frege never gave a systematic account of complex numbers or quaternions. The operation of multiplication was not even described by him.

4 Algebra – the science of pure time

Hamilton read a paper on 'Algebra as the Science of Pure Time' to the Royal Irish Academy in 1835. This was included in his long paper on 'Algebraic Couples' published in the *Transactions of the Royal Irish Academy* in 1837. This is more easily accessible in Volume 3 of his *Mathematical Papers* published by the Cambridge University Press in 1967. Hamilton's theories on algebra as the science of pure time were again given in the preface to *Lectures on Quaternions* with further development in the first 16 sections of that work's preface. The whole preface is included in the same Volume 3 of his *Mathematical Papers*. This is what I will use in giving an account of Hamilton's theories on algebra as the science of pure time. He is concerned to give meaning and interpretation to negative and imaginary numbers. He has already given an account of complex numbers as ordered couples or pairs of real numbers. He is of course familiar with the use of the Argand plane or diagram to explain complex numbers as vectors – i.e. real numbers with direction in two dimensions of space which includes the concept of angles. But he says he feels dissatisfied with any view which does not from the outset give to negative and imaginary numbers a clear interpretation and *meaning*; and he wishes that this should be done, for the square roots of negative numbers, without introducing considerations *so expressly geometrical*, such as those which involve the conception of an *angle*. This will involve giving an explanation and meaning to imaginary numbers using only *one dimension*.

Hamilton then gives a summary of his position and objectives so clearly and explicitly that it must be quoted in full:

It early appeared to me that these ends might be attained by our consenting to regard ALGEBRA as being no mere art nor language, nor *primarily* a Science of Quantity; but rather as the Science of Order in Progression. It is, however, a part of this conception, that the *progression* here spoken of was understood to be *continuous* and *unidimensional*, extending indefinitely *forward* and *backwards*, but not in any *lateral* direction. And although the successive *states* of such progression might (no doubt) be represented by *points upon a line*, yet I thought that their simple *successiveness* was better conceived by comparing them with *moments of time*, divested, however, of a reference to *cause* and *effect*; so that the 'time' here considered might be said to be abstract, ideal or *pure*, like that 'space' which is the object of geometry. In this manner I was led, many years ago, to regard Algebra as the SCIENCE OF PURE TIME: and an essay, containing my views respecting it as such, was published in 1835.[1]

There are at least three important observations to make on this summary of Hamilton's concepts. First, algebra is not primarily a science of quantity. This does not exclude the concept of quantity or measure numbers. The numbers on the unidimensional line are real numbers, measure numbers. Secondly, the concept of order in progression means the numbers on the line are by their very nature ordinal numbers. This is very different from cardinal numbers, which have no ordinal character in themselves unless it is put there subsequently. Thirdly, the unidimensional line of time extends to infinity in both directions, forward and backward: this is the scale of numbers from plus infinity to minus infinity to which Hamilton gave the name scalar. They are scalar numbers – the real numbers – representing the scale of time not length. Time in physics is a scalar quantity, without reference to a direction.

At the end of the passage quoted above Hamilton has a footnote referring to Kant's *Critique of Pure Reason*. He says he was encouraged in these views by remembering some passages in the *Critique* about an a priori science of time, as well as a science of space. He quotes from the 'Transcendental Aesthetic' in German and then gives his own translation:

Time and space are therefore two knowledge-sources from which different synthetic knowledges can be a priori derived, as eminently in reference to the knowledge of space and of its relations a brilliant example is given by pure mathematics. For they are both together [space and time], pure forms of sensuous intuition, and make thereby synthetic propositions possible.

The Critique 7th edition Leipzig 1828.

I understand it to be evident from Hamilton's papers and letters that he developed these ideas about time before he had read the above passage from Kant. But, as Hamilton himself says, he was encouraged to publish the ideas as they were in some way similar to those of Kant. It is most important to emphasise that Kant's synthetic a priori judgements or propositions are true of necessity, i.e. they are axioms in the strict sense of the word – their negation is not possible, non-existent. There is no state of affairs corresponding to their negation.

The development of Hamilton's ideas on time can be shown easily and clearly by simple line diagrams:

Time

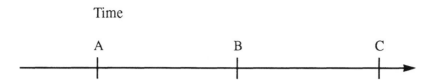

A, B and C are three moments of time or dates on the unidimensional line. A is before B and C is after B. There is an ordinal relation between A, B and C – there is order in the progression of time. You can next consider the duration or quantity in time between A and B and B and C. The dates are ordinal numbers, i.e. scalar numbers. The difference between the dates A and B is a duration. But Hamilton comments that the contrast between the future and the past – B is the future of A and A is the past in relation to B – appears to be even earlier and more fundamental in human thought than that between the great and the little. The next concept is that of steps in time:

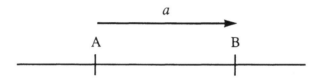

Here, a is the step, duration or quantity of time between the moments or dates A and B. But it is immediately evident that the step a is a vector in the one dimension of time. Complex numbers are vectors in two dimensions, quaternions are vectors in the three dimensions of space and hypercomplex numbers are vectors in n-dimensions, i.e. up to infinite dimensions.

The next stage is the multiplication of the step or vector by –1. This reverses the step or vector to $-a$:

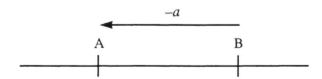

The multiplication of the step or vector $-a$ by –1 reverses the step–vector again – i.e. two successive reversals restore the direction of the vector. Therefore the vector in the one dimension of time has two and only two possible directions, namely forward and backward in time; a is thus a real number which has direction, i.e. a vector. The fact that it has two directions only is still sufficient to give it the character of a vector. To specify the vector in one dimension of time a scalar number is also required, to represent the point from which the vector begins or originates:

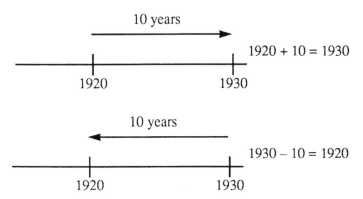

Two numbers are required to specify the vector – you need a scalar number plus a vector number. A complex number considered as a vector in two dimensions of space can have any number of different directions in space. If it is pointed to each degree of a circle, it could point in or have 360 different directions. But the vector in the one dimension of time has two and only two directions, forward and backward. I thought at first that this was analogous to the two directions of intrinsic angular momentum, i.e. spin. Spin has only two directions – left-handed or anticlockwise and right-handed or clockwise. On further consideration this is incorrect use of language. 'Analogous' means partly the same and partly different, whereas there is an exact correlation between the two directions of vectors in one dimension and intrinsic angular momentum or spin.

The next important problem is: how is Hamilton going to give meaning and interpretation to imaginary numbers, i.e. √–1, in the one dimension of time? The answer is given in algebraic form in Section 15 of the preface to his *Lectures on Quaternions*. In Section 16 this explanation is given in words:

In words, if after *reversing* the direction of the second of any two steps, we then transpose them, as to order; thus making the old but reversed second step the *first* of the *new* arrangement, or of the new step-couple; and making, at the same time, the old and unreversed first step the *second* of the same new couple; and if we then repeat this complex process of reversal and transposition, we shall, upon the whole, have *restored* the *order* of the two steps, but have *reversed* the *direction of each*. Now it is the *conceived operator*, in this process of *passing from one pair of steps to another*, which in the system here under consideration was denoted by the celebrated symbol √–1, so often called IMAGINARY. And it is evident that the process thus described has no special reference whatsoever to the notion of space, although it has a reference to the conception of PROGRESSION. The symbol –1 denoted that NEGATIVE UNIT of number, of which the effect as a *factor* was to change a single step (+a) to its own opposite step (–a): and because two such reversals *restore*, therefore (see [10]) the usual algebraic equation $(-1)^2 = +1$ continued to subsist, in this as in other systems. But the symbol $\sqrt{-1}$ *was regarded as not all less real* than those other symbols –1 or +1, although *operating on a different subject*, namely on a pair of steps (a, b) and changing them to a *new pair*, namely the pair (–b +a). And the form of this well known symbol $\sqrt{-1}$, as an *expression* (in the system here described) for what I had previously written as (0,1) and had called (see [15]) the SECONDARY UNIT of number, was justified by showing that the effect of its *operation*, when *twice* performed, *reversed each step* of the pair.[2]

This passage is long and complicated, but if it is illustrated by simple line diagrams the operations are easily demonstrated and a child would have no difficulty in following the various stages of explanation. But the language must be changed in one respect. A 'step' is in fact a vector. It is surprising that Hamilton did not use that term, especially as the passage quoted above forms part of the preface to *Lectures on Quaternions*, a work which is entirely geometrical and involves vectors from the beginning. In his *Elements of Quaternions*, published the year after his death in 1866, the very first line of the work is on the conception of a vector: 'A right line A B, considered as having not only *length*, but also *direction*, is said to be a vector.' Therefore Hamilton's steps in time are vectors in one dimension. Thomas Hankins in his comprehensive biography of Hamilton refers to the steps in time as cardinal numbers which are obtained by counting. The idea that they are vectors in the one dimension of time is completely absent:

It is also proper to call these numbers (or 'multipliers' of the time steps) cardinal numbers, since one may ask 'how many' steps there are between two given moments in time. The answer is one, two, three (and so on), but these cardinal numbers are obtained by counting in progression the steps from the zero moment, and therefore they are dependent on the ordinal relationship of the steps.[3]

Hankins asks how many steps there are (cardinal numbers) between two given moments of time. There are no numbers of steps between two moments of time, there is only one step, a vector – a real number with direction, a measure number of the duration or interval between the two moments or dates in the progression of time which has only one dimension. The concept of cardinal numbers has no relevance here. As Frege has said, cardinal numbers and the real numbers – the measure numbers – belong to completely different domains. Moments of time, i.e. dates, are real numbers – scalar numbers in Hamilton's term – and have no relevance to cardinal numbers, which are used for counting individual objects or members of a class, set or collective. The only concept in common between cardinal numbers and the real numbers or scalar numbers is that of counting. The minutes, hours, days and years are counted, but that counting is totally different from the counting of individual objects.

We must now return to Hamilton's interpretation and meaning of imaginary numbers ($\sqrt{-1}$) in the one dimension of time. The passage quoted earlier giving his explanation in words can now be shown in simple diagrams, beginning with a single vector and its multiplications by -1:

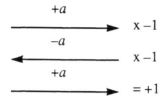

The single vector is reversed by multiplying by -1, and when that operation is repeated the original direction of the single vector is restored. Now we use a couple or pair of vectors and multiply them by -1:

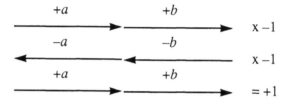

When the pair of vectors is operated on or multiplied by -1 a second time the original direction of the pair of vectors is restored. We now consider the multiplication or operation of $\sqrt{-1}$ on a pair or couple of vectors in one dimension. This operation requires two stages, not one as in operating with -1:

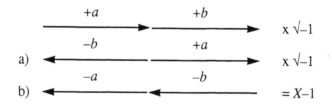

The result of the first operation (a) with $\sqrt{-1}$ is that in effect the second vector $+b$ has been reversed or rotated through $180°$ or π radians and the first vector $+a$ is transposed in its order into second position. The result of the second operation (b) with $X \sqrt{-1}$ is that the same process is repeated – namely that $+a$, which is now the second vector, is rotated through $180°$ – π radians – and $-b$, which is now the first vector, is transposed in its order into second position. The final result is that both vectors are in their original order but both have their directions reversed, i.e. $-a$ and $-b$ – which is the same result as multiplying the pair of vectors by -1, which is what is required to give meaning to $X \sqrt{-1}$ in the one dimension of time. Therefore Hamilton has succeeded in giving a meaning and interpretation to imaginary numbers which does not involve the conception of an angle or geometry or space of two dimensions. The explanation involves only the one dimension of time. The secret of his success is the use of a pair or couple of vectors. In complex numbers $\sqrt{-1}$ operates on a single vector; this involves an ordered pair of real numbers in space of two dimensions. The explanation of $\sqrt{-1}$ in one dimension requires an ordered pair of vectors, i.e. real numbers which have a direction. The concept of order requires two elements. Hamilton calls algebra 'the Science of Order in Progression' and 'the Science of Pure Time'. As stated earlier, it was Hamilton's belief that the contrast between the future and the past was a concept even earlier and more fundamental in human thought than that between the great and the little, i.e. quantity and magnitude.

We must now consider what Hamilton could mean by 'pure time'. In physics time is a scalar quantity or measure. This is Hamilton's own language, the scale of real numbers from $-\infty$ to $+\infty$. This can be shown in a simple diagram of time:

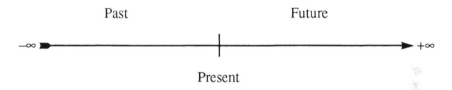

This represents time extending to infinity in both directions, to the past and to the future. The arrows are all pointing towards the future: that is Hamilton's order in progression. As we have seen earlier, this is Hamilton's own conception of time, as expressly given in Section 3 of his preface to *Lectures on Quaternions*:

> this conception [the Science of Order in Progression] that the *progression* here spoken of was understood to be *continuous* and *unidimensional*, extending indefinitely *forward* and *backwards*, but not in any *lateral* direction.

This concept of time having no beginning and no end, i.e. infinite in both directions, is the same as that accepted by most philosophers and scientists. The list includes Plato, Aristotle, Kant, Husserl, Frege, Hamilton and in modern times, for instance, W.H. Newton-Smith of Balliol College, Oxford. Plato's well-known dictum from his *Timaeus* of 'a moving image of eternity' which he called time is very clear and explicit. This is not the place to give exact references to the views of Aristotle, Kant, Husserl or Frege on the eternity of time. Hamilton's views on this subject have already been given. However, Newton-Smith's expression of his own views on time is so clear and explicit and representative of modern thought that it must be given:

> most men in the street, practising physicists and philosophers, have thought with the Platonists that time is *like an unbounded line segment. I will call the topology ascribed to time via this picture the standard topology.* Since this view of time as having the topological properties of being linear, dense (i.e. there is an instant between any pair of distinct instants), non-ending and non beginning, is held generally, it provides a convenient starting point for our investigation.[4]

To condense this into one sentence, time is infinite in both directions. If this proposition is true of necessity, it is an axiom. Using formal logic, which is founded on true premises, i.e. axioms, we can say that the proposition that time has no beginning is logical. Therefore the possibility that time had a beginning is impossible – the concept is non-existent. But it is also possible to make a judgement or proposition that time had a beginning. Again using formal logic, this proposition is an axiom. Therefore the possibility of time having no beginning is an impossibility – it is non-existent. In formal logic you can have only one of the propositions, not both. The judgements based on axioms have only one reference, the True. The human mind, however, can think of both states of affairs – time with a beginning and time with no beginning. The judgements about time have two references – the True and the False in Frege's term as given in the second part of his classic paper *On Meaning and Reference.* There are two states of affairs – what is the case and what is not the case. This involves the explicit rejection of the concept of axioms. To include both references – the True and the False – we must use dialectical logic, which can accommodate two states of affairs – what is the case and what is not the case. Formal logic based on true premises, i.e. axioms, is a theory of identity and its arguments or inferences have validity. Dialectical logic, which has no axioms, is a theory of difference and its arguments or inferences have meaning. In order to have meaning a judgement must have two references, the True and the False. In formal logic to prove a proposition is to infer its validity from true premises, i.e. axioms. The conditions of proofs are two: true propositions, i.e. axioms, and valid arguments. In dialectical logic there are no axioms. To establish meaning you require two judgements: what is the case and what is not the case. The inferences or arguments are then based on the two states of affairs, namely what is the case if the proposition is true and the alternative, what is not the case if it is false.

If time had no beginning, how could you prove this to be the case? If time had a beginning, how could that be proved also? In neither case is proof possible. What is required is for one to study the consequences or inferences from each state of affairs – time with no beginning and time with a beginning. We will now consider time with a beginning by reference to a simple line diagram:

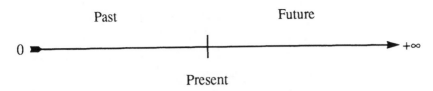

Past   Future

0 ➤━━━━━━━━━━━━━━━━━━━━━━━━━➤ +∞

Present

We now have a scale of time beginning at zero; the number 0 is the origin of the scale. This point of origin provides a perfect reference point for any future date or moment of time. There is a fixed or denumerate number of years from the present to the beginning of time. This is an absolute scale on which negative numbers have no meaning. This is analogous to the Kelvin scale of temperature, whose point of origin or zero is –273° Celsius, i.e. 0° Kelvin, and on which a minus degree of temperature, e.g. –10 Kelvin, has no meaning. With a scale of time which is infinite in the past, on the other hand, there is no such point of reference. The numbers of units of time – seconds, days or years – is infinite by definition. There can be an arbitrary point of reference depending on one's cultural and historical background. For example, the date of the birth of Christ gives AD and BC, while for the Romans the historical date for a reference point was the foundation of the city of Rome in 753 BC – AUC or *anno urbis conditae*. But there is still no absolute reference point as time is infinite in the past.

The next problem to be considered is the arrow of time or time direction – in German *Zeitrichtung*. Chapter 9 of Stephen Hawking's book is entitled 'The Arrow of Time'. The author gives his conclusion on this problem in a few sentences:

> To summarise, the Laws of Science do not distinguish between the forward and backward directions of time. However, there are at least three arrows of time that do distinguish the past from the future. They are the thermodynamic, the direction of time in which disorder increases; the psychological arrow, the direction of time in which we remember the past and not the future; and the cosmological arrow, the direction of time in which the universe expands rather than contracts.[5]

Hawking could have added another, even more obvious arrow of time from biology. Living beings are born, grow, age and die. There is also the evolution of living beings from the simplest forms to higher and higher forms up to human beings. These instances all exhibit a flow of time in one direction – to consider all this in reverse order is an impossibility in reality. The same problem is discussed with equal or even greater clarity in Chapter 7 of Roger Penrose's book *The Emperor's New Mind* entitled 'Cosmology and the Arrow of Time'. Penrose says that there is a conscious awareness of the flow or progression of time – in human experience we are moving forward from a definite past to an uncertain and unknown future:

> Yet physics, as we know it, tells a different story. All the successful equations of

physics are symmetrical in time. They can be used equally well in one direction in time as in the other. The future and the past seem physically to be on an equal footing. Newton's Laws, Hamilton's Equations, Maxwell's Equations, Einstein's General Relativity, Dirac's Equations, Schrödinger's Equation – all remain effectively unaltered if we reverse the direction of time.[6]

The equations of mathematical physics can be expressed in the language of commutability – all the equations commute or are commutative. We can now summarise the presence or absence of an arrow of time in six different categories in tabular form:

The arrow of time

Time direction, or in German Zeitrichtung

Present
1   Conscious human experience and history
2   Biological world
   a) evolution   b) birth   c) growth   d) ageing   e) death
3   The second law of thermodynamics
4   Expansion of the universe

Absent
5   Special theory of relativity – gravitation theory – general theory of relativity
6   Quantum theory

The arrow – i.e. the direction – of time is completely absent from classical mechanics, gravitation theory and also from quantum mechanics. We must ask the question: why is there no arrow of time in these two most fundamental branches of physics? The answer and explanation of this fact is given by G.J. Whitrow in his classic book *The Natural Philosophy of Time*:

Mathematically, the origin – if any – of time is projected to 'minus infinity', which means that in practice it is irrelevant and only time-differences matter. This irrelevance of the origin of time is directly associated with the fact that the time variable does not appear explicitly in the mathematical formulation of the fundamental laws of physics. Indirectly, it is also associated with the fact that the laws of classical mechanics are reversible and do not distinguish between past and future. In classical mechanics there is no special epoch which can serve as a fundamental point of reference with respect to which earlier and later can be distinguished.[7]

The absence of an arrow of time is a consequence of the concept of infinite past time. There is also no fundamental point of reference, because time is infinite in the past. The order of the progression forward or backward makes no difference. Conversely, by a process of negation the presence of an arrow of time is a consequence of the concept of a beginning of time with a perfect point of reference, the origin or beginning. If there is some essential change taking place in the natural world – the cosmos – and extending backwards in time, it must come to a limiting point at the beginning of time. If the universe is expanding in the future, then in the past it is contracting and it reaches a limit at a beginning – a singularity. In this case the order of the progression forward and backward does make a difference. We now have two states of affairs or scenarios which are divided by a negation – they are contradictory, as required by dialectical logic – namely time with an arrow and time with no arrow, and these states of affairs are exactly correlative for time with a beginning and time with no beginning:

Time infinite in past ——————————— no arrow of time
Time with a beginning ————————— an arrow of time

The concept of time direction suggests or, more properly, demands the concept of a vector, or 'step in time' as Hamilton called it. When you have a vector in the one dimension of time, you also require a scalar number to provide the moment or date for the origin or beginning of the vector, as already described.

The concept of the order of the progression in time making no difference or making a difference is an exact correlation of commutative and non-commutative multiplication. If $AB = BA$ the order of symbols representing vectors makes no difference to the result – the equation is equal, it commutes. If $AB \neq BA$ the order of multiplication makes a difference – the equation is not equal, it does not commute.

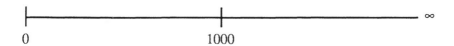

0   1000

As can be seen from the figure above, the step or vector from 0 to 5 years is different from the vector from 1000 years to 1005. This is analogous to the difference in the state of a material from 5° Kelvin to 10° Kelvin and from 200° Kelvin to 205° Kelvin. It is also analogous to the difference in growth in a human being from 5 to 10 years and from 70 to 75 years.

When time is infinite in the past the laws of classical mechanics do not distinguish between past and future – the order forward and backward makes or shows no difference. The final conclusion about these distinctions is that the multiplication of vectors in the one dimension of time with no arrow is commutative. The multiplication of vectors in time with an arrow is non-commutative. Hamilton's thesis that algebra is the science of pure time leads to the question: is there any difference in the algebra between time with an arrow and time with no arrow, i.e. with the order of progression in time making a difference or with no difference? The answer is:

Time	–	No beginning
No arrow of time	–	Algebra commutative

Time	–	With a beginning
Arrow of time	–	Algebra non-commutative

The same concepts apply to the equations in mathematical physics in the examples given earlier by Roger Penrose, e.g. those of Newton, Hamilton, etc.

The equations are equal as a consequence of the absence of an arrow of time – in this case the equations commute. If there was an arrow of time in the physical universe the equations would not be equal – the equations would not commute. In slightly different language the equations would be anticommuting. Therefore the mathematical symbolism of an arrow of time in physics is non-commutative algebra. Earlier I described four different types of non-commutative algebra (see Chapter 3). As already mentioned there are three conditions for non-commutative multiplication:

1 Vectors – real or measure numbers with direction.
2 Rotation.
3 In different dimensions.

I now give a brief summary of the four different non-commutative algebras, beginning with the greatest number of dimensions of space:

1 n-dimensions – Hilbert Space, hypercomplex numbers, or matrix algebras. Involves the symbolism of probability or imprecision. This algebra was used by e.g. Heisenberg in matrix mechanics and in quantum theory.

2 Three dimensions – three vectors
   Involves quaternions, with a special application for describing intrinsic angular momentum or spin with the three directions in space for the three axes of spin. The non-commutative multiplication reverses each axis of spin and consequently the direction of spin in each axis.

3 Two dimensions – complex numbers – one vector
   There are two different states of affairs:
   a) multiplication is commutative with changed angles of vector and no change of length, i.e. Hamilton's versor (change of angle). This generates a closed circle. Left rotation and right rotation are equal.

b) multiplication is non-commutative with a change of angle of the vector (versor) and also a change of length (tensor). This generates a spiral. Left rotation and right rotation are different – they are not equal, which is the non-commutative character of the change – i.e. the orbital angular motion of a body which is in a spiral. Left-handed motion is different from right-handed.

4   One dimension of time
There are three different states of affairs:
a) scalar numbers – real numbers in one dimension – their multiplication is commutative.
b) using a pair or couple of vectors (steps in time as Hamilton called them) with time infinite in the past and no arrow; here the multiplication is commutative.
c) with time having a beginning and therefore with an arrow, the multiplication is non-commutative.

We can combine Hamilton's two concepts of algebra as the science of pure time and algebra as the science of order in progression. There are two possibilities: the order forward and backward makes no difference, or the order forward and backward does make a difference. This is exactly the meaning of commutative and non-commutative multiplication respectively:

$$AB = BA - \text{commutative}$$
$$AB \neq BA - \text{non-commutative}$$

In modern classical mechanics there is no arrow of time, as has already been described in the quotation from Whitrow's book; the order forward and backward is no different. This is why the equations of motion are commutative, the equations commute. If there was an arrow of time, a direction of time – *Zeitrichtung* – the equations of motion would not commute, in other words they would be anticommuting. Therefore the symbolism of an arrow of time in physics is non-commutative algebra in the one dimension of time. The non-commutative algebra used in quantum mechanics is quite different, as has already been described and explained by Sir Edmund Whittaker (see Chapter 3). This is the symbolism of probability or imprecision because of the n-dimensions involved – i.e. Hilbert Space.

The commutative law of multiplication is axiomatic in formal logic. Frege's theory of value-ranges does not apply in this case – the values of the symbols A and B are the same for commutative – $AB = BA$ – as for non-commutative – $AB \neq BA$ – multiplication. Therefore non-commutative multiplication is impossible in formal logic. These contradictory states of affairs can only be accounted for in dialectical logic, i.e. a logic in which judgements or propositions have two references – what is the case and what is not the case

– two states of affairs which are contradictory. This is dialectical logic: it has no axioms, and the most fundamental assertions or judgements are both verifiable and falsifiable. Therefore the question of proof does not arise. Dialectical logic is a theory of meaning.

We must consider the opinions of some philosophers and philosophers of mathematics on the problems of time and numbers. We begin with Aristotle. His famous definition of time is in Book IV of his *Physics*: 'It is clear then that time is the number of movement in respect of before and after.' Aristotle speaks of measuring time by movement. The word 'number' in Greek is *arithmos* – the origin of our word 'arithmetic'. If time is to be measured, it is obvious that the number for time is a measure number – a scalar number. Scientists, especially astronomers, have been measuring time for centuries with greater and greater accuracy up to the present use of atomic clocks. We now turn to St Thomas Aquinas for the account of time in his commentary on the same Book IV of Aristotle's *Physics*:

To perceive motion or time we must take account of *number* i.e. the plurality.

(1) of *cardinal* number, which means simply multitude and which is applicable to non-motion, i.e. to extension;

(2) of *ordinal* number, which gives a determinate succession, a 'before and after'. It is motion that gives the serial numbers. Motions 'something' which time takes over is the ordinal numbers. 'Motion is the actuation of an existent's potency.' Time is not that. 'Therefore it is evident that time is not motion, but takes over from motion the numbering (ordinal) which is peculiar to motion.'

Number in the abstract (as two, three, four) is that *by* which we number. Time is not that. Again, an *actual* multitude is a set of discrete things, as ten men, ten horses. Extent in itself, as a bolt of cloth, is not actual (number) multitude; being a continuum, it is one. The same is true of motion; it is not an actual multitude. Extent and motion are not (actual) number, but they are *numerable*. What time does is to number actually the numerable, motion; just as the draper actually numbers the cloth when he measures it. The numbering is *applied* number in both cases; but the order, succession, direction, is determined in time – measuring; it is not determined in the extent – measuring. That is because time is the measuring of motion, which is numerable, indeed, but numerable ordinally.[8]

Aquinas makes the clear distinction between cardinal numbers and ordinal numbers. Cardinal numbers means multitude, plurality, a set of discrete things, such as ten men and ten horses – Aquinas could be commenting on modern set theory. He refers to measure numbers used for measuring the length of a bolt of cloth. Then he says that the numbers for time are ordinal, successive and have direction: he explicitly states that the numbers for time are measure numbers as well as ordinal. All this is exactly the same as Hamilton's concepts of algebra as the science of pure time and order in progression – which word has the same meaning as 'succession'. Anyone would have to admit it is rather remarkable that St Thomas Aquinas, a

Christian theologian of the thirteenth century, should have concepts of the relation of time and number – ordinal number – identical to but six hundred years prior to that of Hamilton, the greatest mathematician of the nineteenth century. The only concept missing from Aquinas' account is that of Hamilton's steps in time, i.e. vectors in time of one dimension.

We next leap forward to Edmund Husserl's work *Philosophy of Arithmetic*, published in 1891. He refers to 'Sir William Hamilton and his algebra – "The Science of Pure Time" and the "Science of Order in Progression" in English'.[9] In footnote 3 Husserl gives the source of his information, namely a work by Herman Hankel, *Vorlesungen Über die Complexen Zahlen 1867*. Husserl also refers to Hamilton – the mathematician, not the Scottish logician of the same name – in Volume I, Section 70 of his *Logical Investigations*, where he mentions the related theories of W. Rowan Hamilton, which can be readily purged of anything geometric. Husserl was unable to make use of Hamilton's ideas because his own philosophy of arithmetic was based on the cardinal numbers. These numbers have nothing to do with time. Their only possible relationship with time is a psychological one, of the time taken to count the number of individual members of a group, collective or set, such as a farmer counting the number of sheep in his flock and the child in the kindergarten counting the number of marbles in a box. There is in Husserl's work a total absence of any idea that numbers could be ordinal and used for a measure of time. These are the same numbers described by St Thomas Aquinas six hundred years earlier. We now consider Frege's views on time and number. These views are expressed in a few sentences in his *Foundations of Arithmetic*: 'Time is only a psychological necessity for numbering, it has nothing to do with concept of number'[10] and again on the same page: 'Points of time, again, are separated by time intervals, long or short, equal or unequal. All these are relationships which have absolutely nothing to do with numbers as such.' Frege is expressing the same point of view as Husserl, that number has nothing to do with time. The reason is the same as in Husserl's case, namely that his numbers are cardinal numbers, the numbers of axiomatic set theory. There is obviously something seriously inadequate with this theory of time and number. If Frege's theory of numbers was based on the real numbers, measure numbers, then obviously time is measurable: it is a scalar quantity – a real number – in physics. It is not only an important measurable quantity in physics, but the most important measure in physics.

We must next examine Russell's views on time and number, or the lack of them:

Philosophers have usually depreciated time; this is obviously true of Bradley and McTaggert, amongst recent philosophers, and to some extent can be said, to a large degree, of Russell. 'There is some sense,' he had written in *Our Knowledge of the External World*, 'in which time is an important and superficial characteristic of reality. Past and future must be acknowledged to be as real as the present, and a certain emancipation from slavery to time is essential to philosophers' thought.' Any philosopher who approaches philosophy through logic is likely to argue in this way; on the face of it, implication is not a temporal relation and 'truth' as logic understands it is eternal.[11]

This reference by another writer to Russell is so important and remarkable that it is worth consulting Russell's own text to see if he has anything else to add to his extraordinary concept of time. Just after the passage quoted from Passmore Russell says:

A truer image of the world, I think, is obtained by picturing things as entering into the stream of time from an eternal world outside, than from a view which regards time as the devouring tyrant of all that is. Both in thought and feeling, to realise the unimportance of time is the gate of wisdom.[12]

The subtitle of Russell's book is 'As a Field for Scientific Method in Philosophy'. As a scientist and philosopher how could he possibly say that time is unimportant in the external world – so unimportant that to ignore time is the gate to wisdom? Everything in the natural, real world exists in time. In the living world animals are born, grow, age and then die. In evolution all living species develop from simple forms of life to ones of greater organisation, ending in human life. All this takes place as a consequence of the flow of time, the arrow of time – time in one forward direction. In other words, the order of time makes a fundamental difference. If time was reversed all living beings would rise from the dead, grow younger and younger and eventually return to their mother's womb. All this is obviously impossible in reality. Christians believe that Christ rose from the dead, but to think of all human beings and living beings rising from the dead by a pure process of nature is . . . further comment is unnecessary. In physics this unidirectional character of time is totally absent, the order of time makes no difference. Why this should be so is a fundamental problem in physics. What difference would it make in physics if time had an arrow and a direction? All these problems Russell does not even begin to consider. Time is unimportant – to realise this is for him the gate of wisdom. How wrong can you be? He takes it for granted that the world is eternal, that the fact that this is so is axiomatic. But is it true? What difference would it make if it had a beginning? The problem of time and its direction or absence of direction and its measure is perhaps the most fundamental in science and philosophy. But Russell the logician and mathematician has nothing to say about time and its numbering and meaning.

Summary of Hamilton's concept of algebra as the science of pure time and of order in progression

1 Hamilton assumes that time is infinite in both directions in one dimension.

2 Time is considered as both:
   a) infinite in the past
   b) with a beginning.

3 Moments of time – or dates – are points on the unidimensional line of time. Time is order in progression. The moments or dates are ordinal numbers – scalar numbers.

4 Time has a direction – a step in time which is a vector. The vector has only two directions, forward and backward. This is the same as intrinsic angular momentum or spin. It has two directions only: right-handed, clockwise and spin-down, and left-handed, anticlockwise and spin-up.

5 The negative number −1 involves a step in a backward direction – a conjugate vector. If x−1 is repeated, direction is restored to a forward direction.

6 The meaning of $\sqrt{-1}$ is that it operates on a pair or couple of vectors in one dimension in two stages. It reverses and transposes the order of the vectors. When this operation is repeated both vectors are reversed and restored to their original order, the same result as can be gained by multiplying both vectors by −1.

7 The full specification of time requires two numbers:
   a) a scalar number for the date or epoch
   b) a vector or step from that date or epoch. Time requires a scalar and a vector number.

8 Time involves two states of affairs – two scenarios:
   a) Time with no beginning – no point of reference
   b) Time with a beginning. This is an absolute scale beginning with 0 – the origin of the scale.

9 a) Time with no beginning has no arrow of time – the order forward and backward makes no difference. The multiplication of vectors is commutative.
   b) Time with a beginning has an arrow of time – the order forward and backward makes a difference. The multiplication of vectors is non-commutative. The order makes a difference.

10 In their application, the above distinctions correlate with the concept of spin – i.e. intrinsic angular momentum:
   a) Left-handed and right-handed spin are equal – the order of spin makes no difference, and multiplication is commutative.
   b) Left-handed and right-handed spin are not equal – the order of spin makes a difference, and multiplication is non-commutative. This refers to the rate of spin – uniform or not uniform.

11 Using formal logic:
   a) If time is infinite in the past is an axiom, then time with a beginning is impossible – non-existent.
   b) If time with a beginning is an axiom, then the concept of time with no beginning is also impossible – non-existent.

12 If dialectical logic is used, both states of affairs – time with a beginning and time with no beginning – are possible. There is a state of affairs corresponding to each proposition – there are two scenarios. Each can be verifiable and falsifiable – which is a theory of meaning. In order for a proposition to have meaning it must be falsifiable as well as verifiable. This is clearly stated by Ayer in his *Language, Truth and Logic*: 'Since it is only a significant proposition that can be significantly contradicted.'[13]

   Formal logic is based on true premises, i.e. axioms. Proof is based on valid inferences from the axioms. Formal logic is therefore a theory of proof and validity.

   In dialectical logic proof is not involved, only meaning when the proposition has two references, the True and the False. Therefore dialectical logic is a method of discovering what is the truth.

I will conclude with a very apt quotation from Gilbert Ryle:

The story of twentieth century philosophy is very largely the story of this notion of sense or meaning. Meanings (to use a trouble-making plural noun) are what Moore's analyses have been analyses of) meanings are what Russell's logical atoms were atoms of; meanings, in one small sense but not in another, were what Russell's incomplete symbols were bereft of; meanings are what logical considerations prohibit to the antinomy-generating forms of words on which Frege and Russell had tried to found arithmetic; meanings are what the members of the Vienna Circle preferred a general litmus paper for; meanings are what the *Tractatus*, with certain qualifications, denies to the would-be proposition both of Formal logic and philosophy; and yet meanings are just what, in different ways, philosophy and logic are *Ex-Officio about*.[14]

5 Geometry

Euclidean and non-Euclidean geometry – 1

The standard definition of geometry is the science which investigates the properties and relations of magnitudes in space, as lines, surfaces and solids. The universe – the cosmos – exists in space and time. It is usual and universal when writing about the dual concepts of space and time to treat of space first and time second. For example, in Kant's *Critique of Pure Reason*, Section 1 of the 'Transcendental Aesthetic' is on space and Section 2 is on time. But I have done it in the reverse order, with time first and space – geometry – second. This is due of course to the influence of Hamilton's paper on 'Algebra as the Science of Pure Time'. Husserl's philosophy of mathematics is based on his *Philosophy of Arithmetic* of 1891, while Frege's two main works on the philosophy of mathematics are on arithmetic exclusively. There is no philosophy of geometry or space in Frege because their parallel axioms can be denied without contradiction. The axioms of geometry are independent of one another and of the fundamental laws of logic, by which Frege of course means formal logic, which is founded on true premises, i.e. axioms. Can one say the same of the fundamental principles of the science of numbers? Everything would collapse in confusion if one of the principles was denied. Therefore the whole of geometry is excluded because its axioms can be contradicted giving all the systems of non-Euclidean geometry. It seems very strange that Dummett considers Frege the greatest philosopher of mathematics when the whole of geometry is absent from Frege's works, even though geometry is the science of space and the concept of extension which is applicable to the natural real world – the cosmos. Frege always considered the applicability of mathematics of fundamental importance as a science, and not as a mere game with rules and symbols which have no meaning. Frege says that the truths of arithmetic govern the domain of what is countable, and what is countable is individual members of a class or set, namely cardinal numbers, not the real numbers, the measure numbers.

Hilbert's work on the foundations of Euclidean geometry is based on the real number system. Yet with his axiomatisation of geometry and his extreme formalism he deprived geometry of any real meaning. This point of view is well summarised by Mary Tiles in her recent book *Mathematics and the Image of Reason*:

> Hilbert's position was, in a sense, the inverse of Frege's. With his axiomatization of geometry he effectively removed the impulse to treat these axioms as self-evident truths validated by appeal to geometric intuition, or to an intuition of space, for as he emphasized by saying 'it must be possible to replace in all geometric statements the words *point, line, plane* by *table, chair, mug*', there is nothing peculiarly spatial in the conditions laid down by the axioms, they might be satisfied in any domain of objects. Indeed Frege wrote to Hilbert, 'It seems to me that you want to divorce geometry completely from our intuition of space and make it a purely logical discipline, like arithmetic.'[1]

By 'logical' is meant formal logic based on axioms, which is essentially divorced from meaning and the real universe. When Hilbert can say that the point, line and plane can be replaced by table, chair and mug it is obvious that there is something very seriously wrong and unacceptable with his extreme formalist point of view.

We must retain the concept of geometry as the science of space and extension applicable to the real world in which we live. The second part of the word means metric or measure. The concept of extension can be represented by a line extending at least in thought to infinity in both directions:

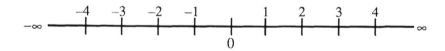

The numbers represent measures of length on a scale, e.g. metres or yards. These are scalar numbers, measure numbers, the real numbers. They are of their very nature ordinal numbers. These are the exact correlation of Hamilton's unidimensional scale of time, the moments or dates of time already described. If space is Euclidean – i.e. flat, with an absence of curvature – the line can be extended conceptually to infinity in both directions giving or generating infinite, or transfinite, ordinal numbers. Since our whole philosophy of mathematics is based exclusively on the real numbers not on the cardinal numbers, the existence of infinite or transfinite cardinal numbers is excluded. The cardinal numbers and real numbers belong to what Frege calls completely disjoint or different domains. Therefore problems or paradoxes involving the correlation of transfinite cardinal numbers and transfinite ordinal numbers cannot arise. The concept of cardinal numbers is specifically and totally excluded: only real numbers – ordinal numbers – are used. These numbers can also be called scalar numbers or measure numbers. The line in space is of only one dimension. The plane is space of two dimensions:

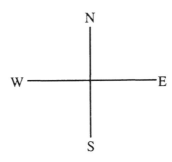

This gives directions in space in two dimensions: east–west and north–South. But the space of the natural real world has three dimensions as well as east–west and north–south. The third dimension is up–down. These are the three directions in the Cartesian coordinate system. The directed lines in this system are vectors, i.e. real numbers which have a direction in two dimensions and in three dimensions. The translatory movement of bodies can be described in the plane with two dimensions, albeit more completely in a plane with three dimensions. But a body which is subject to spin – i.e. intrinsic angular momentum – has no movement of translation – it remains in the same place or location. Even so, for the full description of spin you still require three directions, corresponding to the three dimensions of space, since the axis of spin can have three different directions. These are the units i, j, k of Hamilton's quaternions, as described in Chapter 3:

$ij = +k$ – the axis of spin is upwards
$ji = -k$ – the axis of spin is downwards

The non-commutative multiplication reverses the axis of spin and in consequence the direction of spin. In the earth's orbit around the sun the two motions are combined, namely translatory motion, i.e. orbital angulum momentum, and the rotation or spin, i.e. intrinsic angular momentum. Professor Hawking has very important observations on the physical necessity of a space of three dimensions for gravitation theory:

There would also be problems with more than three space dimensions. The gravitational force between two bodies would decrease more rapidly with distance than it does in three dimensions. In three dimensions, the gravitational force drops to ¼ if one doubles the distance. In four dimensions it drops to ⅛, in five dimensions to ⅟₁₆ and so on. The significance of this is that the orbits of the planets, like the earth, around the sun would be unstable: the least disturbance from a circular orbit (such as would be caused by the gravitational attraction of other planets) would result in the earth spiralling away from or into the sun.[2]

It would appear that three dimensions of space is the correct and only description of the natural real world, at least for gravitation theory. It is difficult to conceive what space of more than three dimensions would be like in reality.

Euclidean and non-Euclidean geometry – 2

In 1733 the mathematician G. Saccheri (1677–1733) published *Euclides ab omni naevo vindicatus*. In this work he attempted to prove that Euclid's system of geometry with its postulate or axiom of parallels was the only one possible in logic and experience. For centuries Euclidean geometry was the paradigm of deductive science, based on the demonstrative premise – what Aristotle called the apodeictic premise, i.e. an axiom – which was a fundamental condition for proof. In his process of proof Saccheri discovered two other types of geometry – both non-Euclidean – without realising the implication of his findings. He was using the concept of formal logic with its foundation on true premises or axioms. In Euclidean geometry the sum of the angles of a triangle is equal to 180°. In the two types of non-Euclidean geometry the sum of the angles of a triangle is less than 180° for negative curvature and greater than 180° for positive curvature. This latter is Riemann's elliptic geometry. In this so-called spherical geometry space is finite but unbounded. Frege had the greatest difficulty in accepting non-Euclidean geometry, or more correctly he was unable to accept it as in any sense true. 'No man can serve two masters. One cannot serve both truth and untruth. If Euclidean geometry is true, then non-Euclidean geometry is false, and if non-Euclidean geometry is true, then Euclidean geometry is false.'[3] He goes on to suggest that non-Euclidean geometry is not a genuine science and compares it to alchemy or astrology.

The whole problem of the two geometries is of the most fundamental importance and consequence for physics and philosophy, especially as non-Euclidean geometry is used in the theory of general relativity. To elucidate the problem I propose to use dialectical logic, not formal logic based on axioms. Dialectical logic has no axioms – its propositions have two references, what is the case and what is not the case. It is a theory of meaning not proof. We can examine what state of affairs corresponds to Euclidean geometry and what state of affairs corresponds to non-Euclidean geometry, by employing exactly the same method used for commutative and non-commutative algebra. Both states of affairs can be accommodated and the consequences of each examined. This involves the study of the meaning of the two categories of geometry, where you have states of affairs which are contradictory – i.e. divided by a negation. The same method – dialectical logic – was used to examine the meaning of time with a beginning and time with no beginning, since the importance and value of dialectical logic is only evident when applied to concepts of the greatest possible generality.

First, we look at the state of affairs corresponding to Euclidean geometry:

EUCLIDEAN GEOMETRY

1   Space is flat, with no curvature.
2   There is an extension of space to infinity.
3   Transfinite ordinal numbers can be applied to an infinity-extended universe.
4   There is only one universe possible.
5   The expansion of the universe or cosmos has no meaning.
6   Any explanation of gravitation as a consequence of the curvature of space is excluded, since space is flat with no curvature.
7   Any concept of a motion of the universe or cosmos from place to place – i.e. translatory motion – has no meaning.
8   Any concept of a rotation of the universe or cosmos has no meaning.

We now give the state of affairs corresponding to non-Euclidean geometry using the same eight categories:

NON-EUCLIDEAN GEOMETRY

1   Space is curved, not flat.
2   The extension of space is finite, but unbounded.
3   Transfinite ordinal numbers have no application as space is finite in extension.
4   As space is finite multiple universes are conceptually possible – up to an infinite number of universes.
5   The expansion of the universe is possible as it is finite in extent.
6   An explanation of gravitation as being due to the curvature of space is possible.
7   A theory of the translatory motion of the universe or cosmos is conceptually possible.
8   A theory of the rotation or spin of the universe or cosmos is also conceptually possible.

We must now comment on the two states of affairs of space – two scenarios – and consider the advantages and disadvantages of each. The great problem is which state of affairs is true of the real universe in which we live?

1 Is space flat or curved?

The supreme example of scientific ignorance is to believe that the earth is flat. To call someone a flat-earther is the greatest possible insult about one's lack of scientific knowledge. Are we to say the same about the assertion that space is flat? If the general theory of relativity is the whole and final truth about the universe, then it is a grave scientific error to maintain that the universe is Euclidean and flat. But the special theory of relativity has no matter, gravitation is absent and space is flat and Euclidean.

2 & 3 Is space infinite and capable of being measured by transfinite numbers, or finite without such numbers?

The human mind can conceive of the universe extending to infinity in all directions, i.e. it is logically possible to have an infinite universe. But if the universe is curved this logical possibility must be denied. The logical and the real do not correspond or correlate. Cantor developed a theory of transfinite or infinite cardinal and ordinal numbers – 'Cantor's paradise', as Hilbert called it – but if space is curved then these numbers have no application in the real curved cosmos which is finite but unbounded. That appears to put a serious boundary or limit to human reason – to the rationality of the universe. But you do not really need Cantor to tell you about infinite numbers. If the universe is infinite in space, then the scalar numbers – real numbers – measuring its extension must be infinite. These numbers are logically possible yet they cannot be applied to the real universe. There is again no correspondence between the logical and the real cosmos. As Chapter 4 explained, the standard topology or theory of time is that it extends to infinity in both directions. Most of the great philosophers and scientists accept the eternity of time. The laws of motion also assume that time can be conceived as extending to infinity in the past, which is why there is no arrow of time in classical physics. If time can be conceived as infinite and the numbers of its measure are the same real numbers, then ordinal numbers can be applied to it. Why must the concept of infinity measured by transfinite ordinal numbers be denied to space? David Hilbert gives a clear account of the issues involved in this important problem in a lecture 'On the Infinite':

> The second place where we encounter the question of whether the infinite is found in nature is in the consideration of the universe as a whole. Here we must consider the expanse of the universe to determine whether it embraces anything infinitely large. But here again modern science, in particular astronomy, has reopened the

question and is endeavouring to solve it, not by the defective means of metaphysical speculations, but by reasons which are based on experiment and on the application of the laws of nature. Here too serious objections against infinity have been found. Euclidean geometry necessarily leads to the postulate that space is infinite. Although Euclidean geometry is indeed a consistent conceptual system, it does not thereby follow that Euclidean geometry actually holds in reality. Whether or not real space is Euclidean can be determined only through observation and experiment. The attempt to prove the infinity of space by pure speculation contains gross errors. From the fact that outside a certain portion of space there is more space, it follows only that space is unbounded, not that it is infinite. Unboundedness and finiteness are compatible. In so called *Elliptical* geometry, mathematical investigation furnishes the natural model of a finite universe. Today the abandonment of Euclidean geometry is no longer merely a mathematical or philosophical speculation but is suggested by considerations which originally had nothing to do with the question of the finiteness of the universe. Einstein has shown that Euclidean geometry must be abandoned. On the basis of his gravitational theory, he deals with cosmological questions and shows that a finite universe is possible. Moreover, all the results of astronomy are perfectly compatible with the postulate that the universe is elliptical.[4]

This passage covers most of the points already made about the infinite extension of the universe and infinite numbers. Hilbert then goes on to say that the universe is finite in two respects: the infinitely small and the infinitely large. He admits that the infinite has a justified place *in our thinking*. It is present in the mathematical theory of analysis where it is a symphony of the infinite. He also says that Cantor's theory of transfinite numbers is the finest product of mathematical genius – the supreme achievement of intellectual human activity – and yet this infinite is nowhere found in reality. Can thought about things be so much different from the reality of things? Can thought be so far removed from reality? The critical problem is clearly stated by Hilbert: the logical and the real do not correspond or correlate. This is unsatisfactory and indeed unacceptable from a philosophical point of view – the logical and the real should correlate. His assertion that the infinite is nowhere to be found in reality is incorrect with respect to time. The concept of time as infinite in the past is fundamental for classical physics, especially for the laws of motion, and for gravitation theory. This is clearly explained in the quotation from Whitrow's *The Natural Philosophy of Time* on page 64. The concept of infinite past time is the explanation for the absence of an arrow of time in classical physics and the reason why the equations of motion are commutative. Hilbert speaks disparagingly of the defective means of metaphysical speculation. This is expressing a loss of power of human reason, even so far as to admit the impotence of reason to discover anything about the nature of the real natural world.

4 Is only one universe possible, or are there multiple universes?

If space is Euclidean it is infinite in extent and logically there can be only one universe. This would appear to have considerable advantages. If you are examining the laws of nature from a philosophical standpoint, there is only one set of the laws of nature as there is only one universe – the real universe. This opens up the possibility of showing that the logical universe and the real universe correspond. But if the universe is non-Euclidean then it is logical that it is finite but unbounded. Therefore multiple universes are conceptually possible up to an infinite number of universes. The laws of nature might apply to one universe and not to other universes. It would then not be possible to argue that the logical universe and the real universe show any correspondence.

5 Is any expansion of the universe possible?

The concept of the expansion of the universe is only possible if space is non-Euclidean as in the general theory of relativity. With Euclidean space the expansion of the universe has no meaning since space is infinite in extent – it is as large as can possibly be conceived. The theory of the expansion of the universe is based on empirical or phenomenological fact, namely the red-shift of the spectra of light from distant galaxies. This explanation is a *spatial* or *geometric* one. The galaxies are alleged to be moving away in space – the Doppler effect. There are two and only two predicates of the universe or cosmos – it has existence in space and time. Therefore there might be another explanation of the red-shift involving some consequence of the passage or flow of time. This would enable the concept of infinite space to be retained.

If the universe is expanding this implies that part of space has no matter or radiation in it – i.e. it is empty or void space. But space should be considered as the locus or place where material reality exists. To have a space with no matter in it seems a contradiction. Going backwards in time the universe is reduced to a point of infinite density or mass – the so-called singularity – with an estimated age of the universe of 15,000,000,000 years. We now have a universe with size of a point and the rest of space empty, which does not appear to make sense or be logical. This is alleged to be the beginning of time, but this cannot be so, since the point mass of infinite density can be conceived to have been in existence from all eternity. Thus, there is no logical necessity why the singularity should be the beginning of time. The laws of nature break down at the singularity, they have no application at that stage.

6 Can gravitation be explained as due to the curvature of space?

The explanation of gravitation as a consequence of the curvature of space obviously requires space to be non-Euclidean. This explanation is again a spatial or geometric one, exactly the same as that required for the expansion of the universe. If the universe is Euclidean and flat some other explanation of gravitation must be found. Again there are only two predicates about the universe or cosmos, namely that it has existence in space and time. If the explanation of gravitation as being due to curved space, i.e. a geometrical interpretation, is excluded the only other possible explanation is that gravitation is due to the action of time, time flowing in one direction – i.e. time with an arrow.

The explanation of the red-shifts of galactic spectra and gravitation as a consequence of the flow of time – an arrow of time, time direction or *Zeitrichtung* – would be a most radical departure from present-day physics and cosmology. It would be a second Copernican Revolution.

7 & 8 Does the universe undergo any translatory motion or rotation?

The concept of the universe itself – rather than its individual constituent stars and planets – being the subject of translatory motion or intrinsic angular momentum – i.e. spin or rotation – is so speculative and unreal that it is not worth any further serious consideration.

We have now discussed the various implications or consequences of the space of the universe being Euclidean or non-Euclidean. This is the same problem as the extension of the universe being infinite or finite. These are two states of affairs – two scenarios – which are contradictory. These two opposed states of affairs can be accommodated in dialectical logic. In axiomatic theory only one theory is possible: whichever of two theories is accepted as true, the other is impossible or non-existent. The only other predicate of the universe is its existence in time. This is a genuine predicate in modern cosmology, as estimates of the age of the universe are given. The concept of time again involves two states of affairs, namely 1) time with a beginning and 2) time with no beginning. In exactly the same way both states of affairs about time can be accommodated in dialectical logic. In axiomatic theory only one theory of time is possible; the other is impossible and unthinkable. I have considered these two theories about the universe separately: time is dealt with in Chapter 4 and space was described earlier in this chapter.

They must now be considered not separately but in conjunction or combination. This is exactly what was done by Kant in his *Critique of Pure Reason* in his examination of the first antinomy of pure reason, and again in his *Prolegomena to any Future Metaphysics*. 'Antinomy' means a theory which leads to contradictory logical conclusions which are not reconcilable. In the *Critique* the first antinomy is in the form of a thesis and its contradiction – the antithesis:

Thesis
The world has a beginning in time and is also limited in regard to space.

Antithesis
The world has no beginning, and no limits in space, but is, in relation both to time and space, infinite.[5]

The two states of affairs can best be set out in simple tabular form, as shown below.

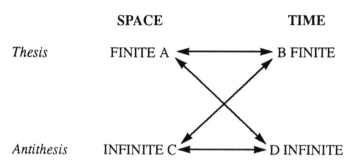

Kant only considers the thesis that space and time are both finite – A B – and the antithesis that space and time are both infinite – C D. But neither of these combinations have any real relevance to cosmology. However, there are two other possible combinations of space–time shown by the crossed arrows A D and C B which Kant did not consider. These combinations have more relevance to cosmology. The first one, A D – that space is finite and time is infinite, i.e. had no beginning – conforms to both modern cosmology and classical physics, i.e. space is finite but unbounded, which is the non-Euclidean geometry of the gravitation theory in general relativity. The other combination, C B – that space is infinite in extent, i.e. Euclidean, and time had a beginning, i.e. is finite in the past – is at least a logical possibility. We now have two states of affairs using the combination of space–time, i.e. two scenarios:

1   Space is finite and time is infinite in the past. This is time with no beginning, therefore time has no arrow as in both the gravitation theory and quantum theory of modern physics. The equations of motion in classical mechanics are commutative, i.e. they commute. Non-Euclidean geometry is required to explain gravitation and the expansion of the universe.

2   Space is infinite and time is finite in the past. This is time with a beginning, therefore time has an arrow and a direction. With space infinite and Euclidean there is only one universe, which is a great advantage from the

logical point of view – there is only one real universe to think about. If space is Euclidean and flat some other explanation of the red-shift of the galactic spectra would have to be found and also another explanation of gravitation – a new theory of gravitation. This explanation could only be provided by the time part of the same combination, namely time with an arrow and a direction. This of course would mean a radical change in modern physics and cosmology.

I must now refer to a most important fact about Kant's arguments for the thesis and antithesis in his theory of time. This is very clearly explained by Stephen Hawking:

> The question of whether the universe had a beginning in time and whether it is limited in space were later extensively examined by the philosopher Immanuel Kant in his monumental (and very obscure) work, *Critique of Pure Reason*, published in 1781. He called these questions antinomies (that is contradictions) of pure reason because he felt there were equally compelling arguments for believing the thesis, that the universe had a beginning, and the antithesis, that it had existed forever. His argument for the thesis was that if the universe did not have a beginning, there would be an infinite period of time before any event, which he considered absurd. The argument for the antithesis was that if the universe had a beginning, there would be an infinite period of time before it, so why should the universe begin at any one particular time? In fact, his case for both the thesis and the antithesis are really the same argument. They are both based on his unspoken assumption that time continues back forever, whether or not the universe had existed forever. As we shall see, the concept of time has no meaning before the beginning of the universe. This was first pointed out by St Augustine, when asked: What did God do before He created the Universe? Augustine didn't reply: He was preparing Hell for people who asked such questions. Instead, he said that time was a property of the universe that God created, and that time did not exist before the beginning of the universe.[6]

We should be very grateful to Hawking for pointing out that Kant assumed or accepted that time extended to infinity in the past. Therefore the thesis and antithesis about time was not an antinomy. There were not two states of affairs which were contradictory. There was only one assertion, namely that time is infinite in the past, which for Kant was an axiom or in his term a synthetic a priori judgement. It is not quite correct to call this an assumption on Kant's part. Twice it is explicitly stated by him that time is infinite in that part of the *Critique* – the 'Transcendental Aesthetic', Section II – on time. The same fact that Kant asserted and accepted that time had no beginning is made by Newton-Smith (1980) in his book *The Structure of Time*, p.101. Kant's theory of time is that it is nothing but the form of our internal intuition. Therefore he is looking at the natural world, the world of experience, through the form or mould of infinite time – i.e. time without an arrow or direction – exactly the same as in modern physics. Kant in his first antinomy is making a judgement, a predicate about the world, i.e. the universe, the cosmos – the world has a beginning in time, and no beginning in time. He has a second judgement about the world as a whole, the universe, the cosmos – space is finite in extension, or infinite in extension. Therefore he has made two judgements or predicates about the whole universe with respect to space and time, each of which is falsified – i.e. there are two states of affairs: space finite and infinite, and time finite and infinite. In modern physical science predicates about the cosmos were only made for the first time with Einstein's general theory of relativity, namely that space is finite but unbounded – a consequence of the use of non-Euclidean geometry. An estimate of the age of the universe is now given by cosmologists. The very name of their branch of study indicates a science of the universe as a whole – but some modern scientists have denied that there are predicates or judgements that can be made about the universe as a whole. One of the most important of these scientists, one of the founders of quantum mechanics – Heisenberg – has expressed his opinion about this problem in his *Physics and Philosophy* (1958) where he says it is important to remember that in natural science we are not interested in the universe as a whole, including ourselves, but we direct our attention instead to some part of the universe and make that the object of our studies. Therefore the object of the scientific study of nature is part of it, not the whole universe or cosmos. One can make the obvious comment 'He would say that, wouldn't he', since Heisenberg was an atomic physicist. Bertrand Russell made important observations about this problem in his introduction to Wittgenstein's *Tractatus*:

> We here touch one instance of Wittgenstein's fundamental thesis, that it is impossible to say anything about the world as a whole, and that whatever can be said has to be about bounded portions of the world.[7]

and again:

> There is no way whatsoever according to him [Wittgenstein] by which we can describe the totality of things that can be named, in other words, the totality of what there is in the world. In order to be able to do this we should have to know of some property which must belong to everything by a logical necessity.[8]

These are also Russell's opinions, especially necessary in view of his logical atomism. The universe is composed of individual units or objects – in his expression property – which must belong to *everything*. However, he cannot deny that the universe exists in space and has extension and also exists in time. But I have already quoted Russell about his theory of the unimportance and irrelevance of time in the natural world. Instead of the universe being a collection of individual objects or elements or members – as in logical atomism – one can think of the universe or cosmos as one reality, one thing, one being – i.e. a monism. This one reality exists in space – it has extension – and in time. It is Being with a capital B, to distinguish it from individual or particular beings such as bricks and stones, planets and stars. These are all part of the one reality, the cosmos. The whole universe is then *one object* of thought. The real numbers – the scalar numbers and measure numbers – are applicable to extension in the one space and to the one time of the universe.

If the philosophy of mathematics is based on cardinal numbers, then these are used for counting the numbers of objects, individuals or members of a group, set or class. As we think of the real universe as an essential unity, one Being, one reality, the concept of a set or class of things or objects is not required – there is only the one thing, the cosmos in space and time. The real number system, the scalar measures, are used or applied to space – i.e. extension – and for time as used by Hamilton in his concept of algebra as the science of pure time (see Chapter 4). The numbers for space and time in geometry are all real numbers, and ordinal numbers by their very essence. The name 'scalar' implies they are on a scale. There is an order in progression which is perhaps more evident in the concept of time. The real numbers of space – i.e. geometry – can have direction, i.e. vectors, in the different numbers of dimensions of space, as described in Chapter 3. Although time has only one dimension it too can have direction – i.e. be a vector, a step in time as Hamilton called it. There are only two possible directions for time, forward and backward, but that is sufficient to apply the concept of vector to time. With spin, or intrinsic angular momentum, there are also only two possible directions: right-handed or clockwise and left-handed or anticlockwise. The atomic physicists have their own terms for the two directions of spin – spin-up and spin-down.

Michael Dummett comments on one of the failures of Frege's philosophy of mathematics:

> These speculations have taken us very far from Frege's work. His failure to make inquiry into the validity of classical logic, as applied to mathematical theories, is the one big lacuna – as opposed to the big error – in his philosophy of mathematics.[9]

Classical logic is based on Aristotle's logic and theory of being or reality. A definition used by scholastic philosophers summarises it in one sentence – logic is the science of the conceptual representation of the real order. But the real order is always of individuals, particular elements or members of a group, set, class or species. The concept is universal, the real is individual. The traditional example given is:

> All men are mortal
> Socrates is a man
> Therefore Socrates is mortal

'All men' is an example of universal quantification. In the theory of the universe as described earlier, the whole universe or cosmos is the subject of predication. The universe is not an individual being or collection of individual beings or objects, as in Russell's logical atomism, but it is one Being, one reality. The use of the concept 'all' is not required, as there is only one thing or reality. This is basically Hegel's philosophy without his idealism. The real universe is existing in space and time. We now have two domains, the logical and the real. The logical is our concept of the universe in extension or space, with two possibilities – the extension is finite or infinite. We also have the logical concept of time, again with two possibilities – time with a beginning and time with no beginning. There are two states of affairs or scenarios:

A	Space – finite	B	Space – infinite
	Time – infinite		Time – finite

The first scenario A, with space finite – i.e. non-Euclidean and curved – and time with no beginning and no arrow, is that of modern physics and cosmology. The second scenario B is a logical concept of the universe or cosmos with space infinite – i.e. flat and Euclidean – and time with a beginning and therefore with an arrow. Using another concept and different words, time with no beginning and no arrow is symmetrical, and forward and backward are no different, whereas time with a beginning and an arrow is non-symmetrical, and forward and backward are different. The two scenarios can be conceived using dialectical logic, in which there are two states of affairs which are contradictory – what is the case and what is not the case. With axiomatic theory only one scenario is possible. If scenario A is axiomatic, scenario B is impossible and non-existent. If scenario B is axiomatic, scenario A is impossible and non-existent. In Hegelian dialectic there are two contradictories, the thesis and the antithesis. These are supposed to be united in a third stage by synthesis. But I would totally reject the concept of the third stage, i.e. synthesis, and retain only the first two stages – the two contradictories what is the case and what is not the case. This is essentially the judgement with two references, the True and the False. But of the two scenarios how do we know or discover which is true and which is false? The answer involves the concept of the coherence theory of truth. Since the universe or cosmos is one reality, theories about it must logically be coherent. The ultimate criterion of coherence theory is that there should be one theory applicable to the science of physics or mathematical physics. This is the goal and ultimate objective of modern physical science – a theory of everything, a unified theory. The two most fundamental theories of physics are gravitation theory and quantum mechanics. Of the two there is no doubt that quantum mechanics is more fundamental. Therefore this should involve the application of quantum theory to the theory of gravitation. Physicists have been attempting to solve this problem – the ultimate goal – although so far without success. I feel convinced that the arrow of time is the key to its solution. If the problem is to be solved one can ask the question: what type of mathematics will be used in the final unification? Formal logic and axiomatic set theory are totally incapable of providing any answer to this question. A logic as described whose subject is not a set of individuals but the universe as a whole – one reality – can be called ontologic – i.e. a logic of being, of the cosmos existing in space and time. A logical universe is one which is coherent and rational. The logical – the concept of the universe – and the real universe should correspond or correlate. In Aristotelian philosophy the concept of a logical universe has no meaning because everything real is an individual object. The logical concept is a universal concept, whereas the real is individual, a purely contingent factual reality, which is not fundamentally related to time. Individuals come to be and pass away. Time is both before their existence and after they cease to exist. That is why one can say that existence is not a predicate because the existent being one is referring to is an individual. But the existence of the universe – the cosmos as a whole, the one reality – is a predicate. The existence of the whole natural world is taken for granted; it is the object of all the sciences, physics, biology and the human sciences.

Kant's philosophy of mathematical physics

We now examine briefly Kant's philosophy of mathematical physics in the following five domains:

1 Kant's theory of judgement
2 Space and time
3 The Copernican Revolution
4 Existence and predication
5 The ontological argument for the existence of God

In each domain I will state how he agrees or does not agree with my own points of view.

1 Kant's theory of judgement

Kant's fundamental theory of judgement is based on the synthetic a priori judgements. These judgements are true of necessity because of their a priori character. Therefore they are axioms. They are axioms in the truest sense in that their negation is not possible, it is non-existent – there is nothing corresponding to their negation. These judgements are augmentative; an example Kant gives is that of the conservation laws. His analytic a priori

87

judgements he calls explicative. They are also true of necessity because they are a priori; their negation is not possible as they are true of necessity, i.e. axioms. In dialectical logic – which I am using – the judgements have two references, the True and the False; there are two states of affairs, what is the case and what is not the case. Therefore there are no axioms because everything is falsifiable. There is a state of affairs corresponding to the judgement both being true and being false.

2 Space and time

A – Space
In Kant's definition, geometry is a science which determines the properties of space. The principles of geometry are always apodeictic – i.e. true of necessity. Here Kant is referring of course to Euclidean geometry. According to Kant, space does not represent any property of objects in themselves. Space is nothing but the form of all phenomena of the external sense; it is a subjective condition.

In contrast I have to reject the concept of space as subjective. Geometry is the science of the space of the real natural world, the universe or cosmos. The concept of space is retained but its character is changed from subjective to objective. For Kant geometry is a synthetical science a priori – i.e. Euclidean geometry is axiomatic. Again I reject Kant's ideas here: there are two possible geometries using dialectical logic – Euclidean and non-Euclidean. Again there are no axioms: the two types of geometry are possible as concepts – two states of affairs – therefore space is an objective property or predicate of the real universe but there are two possible geometries of this space – Euclidean and non-Euclidean.

B – Time
Time for Kant is the form of our sensuous intuition. It is a subjective condition of our human intuition. Kant explicitly rejects the notion that time has any objective reality, that it is the property of anything in reality. Time has one dimension and different times are successive. Twice he explicitly states that time is infinite and can be represented by a line progressing to infinity, meaning of course in the past. Therefore time is one-dimensional – i.e. successive – infinite in the past, and subjective. It is not the property or predicate of the real natural world.

The fact that time is infinite is a synthetic a priori judgement means that the concept of time with a beginning is impossible, it is non-existent. Its extension to infinity in the past is an axiom. In my philosophy the subjective character of time must be totally rejected. Time is a predicate of the real natural world, the cosmos. Time is the measure of motion or change in the real world. I accept Kant's one-dimensional character of time and also its successiveness. Using dialectical logic again, the judgement of time has two references: it is infinite in the past, i.e. no beginning, or it has a beginning. Kant then accepts as a priori judgements the concepts that space is Euclidean and therefore infinite in extent and that time is infinite in the past. Space and time as both infinite are therefore axioms. Therefore these judgements are not antinomies, i.e. contradictions which cannot be reconciled. But it is possible to think of Euclidean space as finite in extent. That means there is space with no matter or reality in it, empty space or void space. This would seem to be a logical contradiction – i.e. space with nothing in it. Space should be the locus or place where material reality exists. The same problem applies to time. It is possible to think of time as extending to infinity in the past and the universe as having a beginning in time, as described in biblical revelation. This is how Issac Barrow and Newton were able to reconcile the Christian belief of the temporal origin of the universe with the infinite past time of their mathematical physics. It entails a time from all eternity before the universe was created at the beginning. However, this means time with no universe or no existing reality, which is a contradiction and completely unacceptable. Time is the measure of motion in the real universe, therefore time before a real universe existed has no meaning. But a quite different state of affairs is the possibility that the real universe and time had a simultaneous beginning.

Kant conceives of motion as the change of place of a body in time. This is a combination of space and time. But he has no reference to the motion of spin or intrinsic angular momentum – i.e. a motion without any change of place.

3 The Copernican Revolution

Kant's use of the analogy of this revolution is described in the preface of the second edition of the *First Critique* It is fundamental to understanding his whole philosophical standpoint and must be quoted in full:

It has hitherto been assumed that our cognition must conform to the objects; but all attempts to ascertain anything about these objects a priori, by means of conceptions, and thus extend the range of our knowledge, have been rendered abortive by this assumption. Let us then make the experiment whether we may not be more successful in metaphysics, if we assume that the objects must conform to our cognition. This appears, at all events, to accord better with the possibility of our gaining the end we have in view, that is to say, of arriving at the cognition of objects a priori, of determining something with respect to these, before they are given to us. We here propose to do just what COPERNICUS did in attempting to explain the celestial movements. When he found that he could make no progress by assuming that all the heavenly bodies revolved around the spectator, he reversed the process, and tried the experiment of assuming that the spectator revolved, while the stars remained at rest. We may make the same experiment with regard to the intuition of objects. If the intuition must conform to the nature of the objects, I do not see how we can know anything of them a priori. If on the other hand the object conforms to the nature of our faculty of intuition, I can easily conceive the possibility of such a priori knowledge.[10]

In this passage Kant is assuming that reality is composed of objects, particular individual objects. But my whole philosophy of physics is based on the conception that reality – the natural world, the cosmos – is *one object*, one reality, existing in space and time. There are no objects in the plural, there is only one object – the cosmos – one reality. This makes it easier to carry out Kant's experiment or suggestion that the one object – the cosmos – might conform or correlate with our conception of it as existing in space and time. For Kant these latter two concepts were both infinite of necessity; they were both synthetic judgements a priori, i.e., they were axioms.

It is interesting to consider that although the Copernican Revolution displaced the earth from being thought of as the centre of the universe, human beings still remained in the centre of the universe as thinking beings and as observers. This is clearly seen in the role of the observer with respect to translatory motion in the theory of relativity and in the act of measurement in quantum mechanics. The Copernican Revolution resulted in the transfer of the earth from the centre of the universe where it was at rest in two respects – i.e. being thought of as lacking any translatory motion and intrinsic angular momentum or spin – to an earth with an orbital motion around the sun and also having spin. Even so, Newton's theory of gravitation is entirely concerned with the orbital motion of the earth around the sun, while its spin – intrinsic angular momentum – is completely ignored and is not part of his theory of gravitation. Exactly the same applies to Einstein's general theory of relativity – the spin of the earth is no part of the theory, it is completely absent from it. Yet spin, or intrinsic angular momentum, is an essential and funda-mental concept in quantum mechanics.

4 Existence is not a predicate

It is perfectly clear that the existence of particular, individual objects is not a predicate. These are the same objects already mentioned in the passage from Kant quoted above. The problem of existence is directly related to time. If a house was built in 1920 it had no existence before 1920. My dog Prince is three years old, therefore four years ago he had no existence. But if the whole universe is one reality, one Being and not a collection of individual objects, then its existence is a predicate. The natural world in which we live and which scientists – especially astronomers – have been studying for centuries has existence. Its existence is a predicate: it has existence in space and time. It has existence before the existence of any human beings. Time is a predicate of the whole universe or cosmos. Time is not a predicate of individual beings. Individual beings come into existence in time, and later cease to exist. The whole universe has existence in time, and cosmologists can give an estimate of the age of the universe. The problem of whether the universe exists from all eternity or has a beginning is a scientific and philosophical one.

5 Ontological argument for the existence of God

St Anselm (1033–1109) used this argument to demonstrate the existence of God. What he meant by God was 'that than which nothing greater can be conceived'. This argument was rejected by Kant and St Thomas Aquinas, because you cannot argue from the mere concept of a being to its actual existence. But to my mind the ontological argument should not be applied to the possible existence of God, but instead to the existence of the universe – the cosmos. If we substitute the universe – the cosmos – for 'God', the argument then is as follows: the universe – the cosmos – is 'that than which nothing greater can be conceived'. The greatest universe the mind can conceive is a universe of infinite extension, which is a Euclidean one – with flat space. The advantages of a Euclidean space, i.e. of infinite extent, have already been described. If space is infinite in extent there is only one universe, which is a special advantage from a logical point of view. Transfinite ordinal numbers thus have an application in the real universe. If the universe is infinite in extent the expansion of the universe has no meaning, therefore another explanation of the red-shift of galactic spectra must be provided. If it is not due to a spatial or geometrical phenomenon, the only other possible explanation is one involving time – the flow of time in one direction, i.e. the arrow of time. The same problem arises with the explanation of the force of gravitation. If it is not due to the curvature of space – i.e. a geometric explanation – the only other possibility is that it is a consequence of the flow of time with direction, the arrow of time – i.e. asymmetric time.

The following is a summary in tabular form of Kant's philosophy of physics and my own.

KANT	MY PHILOSOPHY
1 Synthetic a priori judgement – axioms	1 Dialectical logic – no axioms Judgements with two references – the True and the False

2 Space and time both subjective
One scenario, which is axiomatic
Space is Euclidean and infinite
Time is infinite
	2 Space and time both objective
	Two scenarios
	a) Space is finite and non-Euclidean
	  Time has no beginning
	b) Space is Euclidean and infinite
	  Time has a beginning

3 Copernican Revolution Objects conform to the mind	3 Only one object, the real universe or cosmos Real universe – a unity should conform to our concept of it

KANT	MY PHILOSOPHY
4 Existence (of individual objects) not a predicate	4 Existence of the one real universe is a predicate
5 Ontological argument for existence of God rejected	5 Ontological arguments accepted – but they apply not to God but to the one real universe – the cosmos

Onto-logic (with a hyphen) is logic whose subject is the real universe – the cosmos existing in space and time. The numbers used for the measuring of space – the scalar numbers of length or extension or the real numbers – are the same real numbers as used for the measuring of time – again scalar numbers. The real numbers used for space have direction – i.e. they are vectors in space of various dimensions. The same real numbers used for time also have direction – i.e. they are steps in time, or vectors in the one dimension of time, as described by Hamilton (see Chapters 3 and 4).

Formal logic has no application whatever to the real universe. One definition of formal logic is: the analysis, without regard to meaning or content, of the patterns of reasoning by which conclusions are validly derived from sets of premises. The premises must be true, i.e. axioms whose negation is impossible and non-existent. This is a theory of validity and proof, not of meaning.

The following is Mary Tiles' account of mathematical formalism:

If mathematics is just a formula game then there is no point in demanding significance of mathematical work, just invent and play with formal systems. It is a recipe for a kind of freedom, a freedom from responsibility, which can create empty formalisms. If you think that is all you should be doing, then that may very well be all you do. Outside of mathematics it has the effect of investing computers with power of reason and of divesting reason of power to intervene in distinctively human affairs of ethics, politics and daily life. Reason bound by formal rules is tied within language, within cultures, stands in opposition to freedom and creativity. Gödel's theorem was seen as a demonstration that the human mind is not a machine, was taken as proof of the limits of reason. Having put reason in formal chains it was now found to be impotent. Western philosophy as the way of reason, of logos could be renunciated now that it had deconstructed itself.[11]

It is very encouraging that a woman should be the champion of 'Mathematics as the Image of Reason'.

Summary

Geometry – Euclidean and non-Euclidean

Logically there are only two possible kinds of space:

1   Euclidean space is infinite in extension.
2   Non-Euclidean space is finite in extension but unbounded.

But this is incorrect in formal logic, which is based on true premises, i.e. axioms. The latter are judgements which are true of necessity; they are judgements which have only one reference, the True. In dialectical logic the judgements have two references – not true *or* false but more correctly true *and* false, i.e. two states of affairs: what is the case and what is not the case – thus space can be infinite in extension and finite in extension. Both states of affairs with respect to extension can be accommodated in dialectical logic. But in formal logic based on axioms only one state of affairs is possible – space is either infinite in extension – Euclidean geometry – or finite but unbounded – non-Euclidean geometry. This is why Frege could not accept non-Euclidean geometry in his philosophy of mathematics. Euclidean geometry was founded on axioms, which by definition are true of necessity. Therefore Frege was forced to regard non-Euclidean geometry as not only false but also unscientific, like astrology or alchemy, which are completely fictitious sciences. But you cannot have a philosophy of mathematics without any consideration of geometry and a theory of space and its extension and the number of dimensions of space.

The theory of geometry as developed in this present chapter is placed after the theory of time as described in the previous chapter on Hamilton's concepts of algebra as the science of pure time. There the same two states of affairs are used – time with no beginning and no arrow; and time with a beginning and with an arrow, i.e. time direction. The two states of affairs can be accommodated in dialectical logic but not in formal logic based on axioms. The two concepts – space and time – can be considered in conjunction as in Kant's first antinomies. These antinomies can be expressed in a simple diagram:

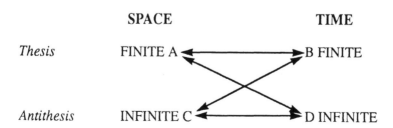

	SPACE	TIME
Thesis	FINITE A	B FINITE
Antithesis	INFINITE C	D INFINITE

Kant's cosmology follows C–D: space is Euclidean and infinite in extension, and time is infinite in the past – i.e. there is no arrow of time. The equations of motion commute.

The general theory of relativity follows A–D: space is finite but unbounded, i.e. non-Euclidean, and time is infinite in the past – i.e. there is no beginning, no arrow of time. The equations of motion commute.

The logical universe theory follows C–B: space is Euclidean and infinite in extension, and time is finite in the past with a beginning and an arrow of time – a direction. The equations of motion do not commute – they are anti-commuting.

If space is finite but unbounded – i.e. non-Euclidean – multiple universes are possible, therefore any concept of a logical universe is excluded. If space is infinite – i.e. Euclidean – there is only one universe to consider, a great advantage since it makes possible a conception of the universe as logical. If the universe is Euclidean it would mean a radical rejection of the general theory of relativity – this would be a second Copernican Revolution. The explanation of gravitation and the red-shift of galactic spectra can no longer be a spatial and geometric one. Another explanation must be provided. They could be explained as a consequence of the flow of time in one direction, i.e. the arrow of time.

6 Measurement and numbers

The first problem in this aspect of the philosophy of mathematics is to consider what is to be measured. The principal measures are length or extension in space, time, angle, temperature and mass. There are also many other measures, e.g. those for volume or capacity and electric charge. The numbers expressing these measures are scalar numbers, the real numbers; by their very nature the numbers on a scale are ordinal numbers. The numbers on a scale – for example for time – can be considered to extend to infinity in both directions. This was Hamilton's original concept of a scalar number. Another term for them is measure numbers: they measure magnitudes or quantities. The number 0 is normally the point of origin of the scale. On a tape measure for length the number 0 is the beginning of the scale. Similarly, on the Celsius scale of temperature 0 is the freezing point of water, and –10° is 10° below the freezing point of water. But on the Kelvin scale of temperature there is an absolute scale – –273°C – below which any temperature is non-existent. The temperature –10° Kelvin has no meaning since 0° Kelvin is the origin of an absolute scale. If time had a beginning the number 0 would be the point of origin of an absolute scale of time.

The number one is the basic unit of quantity or measure: the metre, the yard, the second. Each measure has different quantities or ratios: 12 inches or one foot, three feet or one yard, one metre or 100 centimetres. These numbers are ratios, fixed by various rules and conventions. There is one measure which is quite different from all other measures, namely that of an angle, which is so fundamental for mathematics and physics. Frege calls it a cyclical measure. A circle has 360°. A right angle is a quarter of that, i.e. 90°. In mathematics a more fundamental measure of angles is used, namely the radian. This is the angle between two radii that cut off at the circumference of a circle an arc equal in length to the radius. Therefore 2π radians = 360°; π radians = 180°; ½ radians = 90°. These measures of angles are quite independent of any convention such as the number 360° for a circle. The concept of counting can be applied to the process of measuring. But in many cases the use of counting is not necessary. If you have a foot rule and want to measure the length of a small box (less than a foot long) you read off the length on the ruler; no counting is necessary. But if you want to measure the length of a room and only have a foot rule, you must count the number of lengths of ruler used. The last fraction of the length must be read off from the ruler. If you want to buy 3½ metres of cloth the shopkeeper who has a metre length on the counter, counts three lengths of the metre measured from the roll or bale of cloth and reads off the last measure of the fraction of the metre, namely 50 cm. If you want to measure the length of a garden and have no measuring tape the approximate length can be found by counting the number of paces, the average pace being about one yard. For the measurement of a large area such as a field the process of counting will be necessary. A chain of 22 yards could be used, the number of lengths of the chain used being counted. For measurement of weight counting is usually not necessary: you can read off the weight directly from the scales – the apparatus from which the very name scalar number derives. But if you only have a balance with one-pound weights, you count the number of weights needed to balance the goods that are to be weighed. The use of counting for the measurement of time is still more obvious – you count the minutes, the hours, the days. The numbers on a clock face or a calendar are scalar numbers for the measurement of time. Heidegger in Section 81 of his *Being and Time* says that 'time is that which is counted'. He gives Aristotle's definition of time: For this is time; that which is counted in the movement which we encounter in the measurement which we encounter within the horizon of the earlier and later. Aristotle uses the word 'counted', but the original Greek is *Arithmos* – 'number' of movement. That number is a scalar number, a number that is counted. Heidegger also makes the important observation that the measurement of time gives it a marked public character. If the concept of time is a subjective one, the possibility of its measurement is removed or excluded – which is an unacceptable state of affairs as time in fact has been measured for many centuries with greater and greater accuracy.

All measurement requires a method of standardisation, otherwise the units of measure will not be equal. There should be a one-to-one correspondence between the measure and the standard. When you buy a new foot rule or a metre rod you expect that it is an accurate one. The factory that made it will have a standard measure to ensure absolute accuracy. All rulers made in the factory will show a one-to-one correspondence between their scales. The same measure, e.g. of length, mass or temperature, can have different scales of measure: length has yards and metres; weight has pounds and kilograms, and temperature has Celsius and Fahrenheit. There are fixed ratios for the conversion of one scale of measure to the other. Every local authority has a department of weights and measures to ensure the correct standards, i.e. using the concept of one-to-one correspondence between the standard and each individual scales or measure. The measurement of time has very special problems and different scales, although with scientific advances the measurement has become more accurate. In the past there was particular difficulty in constructing accurate clocks. Details of these methods will be described later, but for now there remains the problem of which of the two most fundamental measures, i.e. length or time, is the primary standard.

It might be thought that modern science was essential for providing adequate standards of measurement. But long before modern scientific advances ancient civilisations had detailed and elaborate standards of measurement. Any commentary or encyclopaedia of the Bible will give details of measurement in Old Testament and New Testament times. In *A Catholic Commentary on Holy Scriptures*[1] there is a chapter on 'Measures, Weights, Money and Time'. The Hebrew measures of length, like all similar measures, are derived from the human body: the cubit, the palm (or hand) and the finger. In New Testament times the Greek cubit of almost exactly 18 inches was used. These measures and the ones for capacity, money and time were all counting numbers – scalar numbers, the real numbers.

The late Professor O.A.W. Dilke has published a most valuable small book on measurement in past times, entitled *Mathematics and Measurement*.[2] The name of the book is most significant, since it is an identification of mathematics and measurement – again the scalar numbers, counting numbers. It has an extensive bibliography and numerous references to the history of science and mathematics, particularly to that of the early period, especially Egypt, Greece and Rome. The author, who was Professor of Latin at the University of Leeds, has also written a book on the Roman land surveyors, based on a collection of manuals of various dates, the *Corpus Agrimensorum*. Such work was carried out by *agrimensores*, literally 'land measurers'. In the Agora at Athens there were official weights and measures inspectors (*metronomoi*). The book contains photographs of a Roman bronze set-square, dividers, a ruler and plumb-bob. There are also photographs of an Egyptian and a Roman weighing scale. The smallest Roman measurement, like the smallest Greek one, was a finger-breadth (*digitus*) – four of these finger-breadths formed a palm or hand. The latter measure is still used for measuring the height of horses to this day. There is even a legacy of Roman land surveying techniques which has survived to the twentieth century. The surveyor's pole was called *pertica* or *decempeda* and its length, as implied in the latter name, was ten Roman feet (approximately 2.96m). The English measure was 'rod, pole or perch' and this last name is derived from *pertica*.

All the numbers used in measurement are scalar numbers, the real numbers of mathematics. Each of them is an ordinal number by the very fact that they are on a scale, thus their ordinal character is of their very essence. The cardinal numbers of axiomatic set theory are completely different. They are the numbers of collections of things, objects or members. There are numerous other words for the same concept: aggregates, groups, sets, classes, etc. of individual objects. They are the answer to the question: how many objects are there? Cardinal numbers have no ordinal character in themselves unless it is deliberately put there. Even when they are put in order they are totally different from the scalar numbers – the measure numbers. The 60° on a thermometer, the number 50 on a tape measure, the number 190 on a weighing scales are all scalar numbers; they have no relationship to groups of objects or sets or aggregates or collections. They are completely different from the cardinal numbers. The use of counting is most obvious with the cardinal numbers – you are answering the question how many objects there are. A child counts the number of marbles in a box, the farmer counts the number of his cows in the field. The failure clearly to distinguish the two uses of counting – one for individual objects or members of a class, set or collection and the other for the number on a scale, using the measure or scalar numbers – has 'led the learned astray', as Frege said. The word 'cardinal' means a hinge; everything hinges on such numbers. Thus for Frege they were the most important numbers. In my view the real numbers – the measure numbers – should be the 'cardinal' numbers, since the etymological use of the word 'real' indicates that they are the most important. My whole philosophy of mathematics is based on the real numbers – the scalar or measure numbers – exclusively.

Systems of philosophy

In the last century many philosophers with a special interest in the human studies, e.g. history, art, moral theory, named their subject *Geisteswissenschaften* – the mental sciences or cultural sciences. They distinguished it from *Naturwissenschaft* – natural science which included both the biological sciences and the physical sciences. Such thinkers included Windleband, Rickert and Dilthey and in this century Hans Georg Gadamer. The major work of many other philosophers is based primarily on the study of human beings. Hume's *A Treatise of Human Nature* by its title indicates its subject matter. Husserl's *Phenomenology* is the study of human consciousness. In Heidegger's major work *Being and Time* the 'being' of the title is *Dasein* – the human being, the being who asks the question what is the meaning of being? For Aristotle the primary existent beings, the living beings of biology, were individuals – they are obviously separate objects of study. The same of course applies to human studies – they are also individual beings, separate objects of study. In modern times, however, since the great development of the physical sciences beginning with Copernicus and Galileo, through

Newton and up to Einstein's theory of relativity and quantum theory and cosmology, the fundamental science – physics – is based on the study of the inanimate physical world, all theories of which are expressed mathematically. The whole physical universe – the cosmos – must be considered as one reality, one Being, the cosmos existing in space and time. There is no essential unity – organic unity – in physics, e.g. of objects, electrons, atoms, molecules, planets and stars. They are all part of the one reality of physical nature whose linking phenomenon is electromagnetic radiation. Therefore natural science must be divided into two sciences – the physical sciences and biology. The human sciences – *Geisteswissenschaften* – are already separated from natural science, so as a consequence we have three separate sciences:

1 The physical sciences – mathematical physics.
2 Biology – living organisms.
3 The human sciences – history, art, moral theory, study of religion, human action, etc.

These three domains of study correspond to Husserl's system of regional categories based on regional axioms, as described in Section 16 of his *Ideas I*.

As we have just seen, there is a fundamental difference between physical science and cosmology and biology and the human sciences. The latter two, biology and the human sciences, are based on individuals which can exist in groups, classes or species. In physical science there is no individuality; there is only one reality existing in space, i.e. extension, and time, as described by Kant in the 'Transcendental Aesthetic' of his *Critique of Pure Reason*. In Hilbert's *Philosophy of Mathematics* (1983), edited by Benacerraf and Putnan, the second of the book's four parts is 'The Existence of Mathematical Objects'. In Michael Dummett's book *Frege – Philosophy of Mathematics*, Chapter 24 deals with 'The Problem of Mathematical Objects'. But as already described we are considering the whole natural physical world – the cosmos as one reality, one thing, one Being – there are no objects in the plural, only one object. This has fundamental consequences for our concept of number. As Frege says, cardinal numbers answer the question, how many objects of a given kind are there? Whereas the real numbers can be regarded as measurement numbers which state how large a quantity is as compared with a unit quantity.

Cardinal numbers are the numbers used for counting the individual members of a set, group, class or aggregate. But as the physical world is one reality these cardinal numbers cannot be used. We use instead the real number system – the scalar numbers, measure numbers, ordinal numbers. Cardinal numbers and set theory are not used.

The change from reality as a collection or aggregate or class of individuals to reality as one thing, one Being, one object – the cosmos – entails a radical change in the conception of logic. The classical logic is based on classes of individuals. The scholastics define logic as the science which treats of the conceptual representation of the real order. But the real order for Aristotle and all the scholastic philosophers is individual. The study of reality – the cosmos – does not deal with thoughts, as does logic, but with things, i.e. not with the conceptual order but with the real order, meaning collections of individuals. Logic on the other hand deals with the conceptual order, with thoughts. Its conclusions do not relate to things, but to the way in which the mind represents things. The word 'things' is in the plural, meaning classes or collections or sets of individual objects or beings. In this theory of logic the concepts of a logical universe which is a collection of individual objects is meaningless and impossible.

If the universe – the cosmos – is one reality with existence in space and time, it is open to the possibility of one theory of change or motion applying to the one universe. This is not only a possibility but a logical necessity, i.e. one theory is sufficient to describe it, or in other words the laws of nature must be coherent. The ultimate coherence is unity: the laws should be reduced to one law, the most fundamental one describing motion in the cosmos. If our concept of the fundamental law is correct it must correspond or correlate with the motion or change in the real universe which is one reality; with this theory of logic there is a possibility that the real universe and our conception of it as expressed in a fundamental law of nature might correlate or correspond. This logic of the whole universe which is one reality is basically the logic of Hegel and the other idealists Bradley and Bosanquet. Their idealism is of course rejected, but the concept of the essential unity of the cosmos is retained. We now have two domains, the logical and the real, and a possible correlation between the two. Scientists, especially astronomers have been studying and observing the natural world for centuries. The existence of the universe is a predicate. The existence of individual beings, especially living organisms and human beings, is obviously not a predicate: they come to be, grow, age and pass away with the progression of time. The universe is a Being – one Being. To be is to exist in time, and time can have a beginning or no beginning and consequently a direction, an arrow, or no arrow, i.e. time is asymmetric or symmetric. Each of these states of affairs can have physical correlates. This is the thesis and antithesis of the Hegelians – the dialectic, two states of affairs which are divided by a negation. The further stage of synthesis is not used: we use only the thesis and antithesis, what is the case and what is not the case, i.e. in effect the judgement which has two references, the True and the False. No use will be made of the stage or process of synthesis of the contradictory judgements. This logic is onto-logic (with a hyphen), the logic of being. The 'being' of the natural world – the cosmos – is in time, therefore this onto-logic is linked to or based on time. The fact that modern cosmologists give an age of the universe and express opinions about the beginning of the universe is evidence of the reality of time. The idealists have traditionally attempted to deny the reality of time, which of course for the physicist and especially for astronomers is completely unacceptable. A view of time which is confined to a subjective character – such as Kant's and Husserl's work on internal time-consciousness – must lead and does lead to the denial of the concept of public time, time as a measure of motion and change. This public time has been measured by scientists, especially astronomers, for centuries, with greater and greater accuracy. The more recent use of atomic clocks gives the greatest possible accuracy.

To return to Michael Dummett's book *Frege – Philosophy of Mathematics*, the author states in the first sentence of his chapter on 'The Problem of Mathematical Objects' that:

> The logicist thesis failed because of its inability to justify the existence of mathematical objects satisfying the axioms of the theories of natural numbers and of real number. [3]

The logicist is of course using formal logic, based primarily on Aristotelian logic. The axioms are based on true premises, i.e. judgements which have one reference only, the True, and whose negation is non-existent. The application of mathematics is to the one real universe, the cosmos existing in space and time – i.e. there is only one object, the one reality. The real numbers are used or applied to the measurement of space – i.e. extension – and time. They are scalar numbers. The logic used is dialectical, i.e. with judgements which have two references, the True and the False, two states of affairs, what is the case and what is not the case. This logic and theory of reality provides a better foundation for the philosophy of mathematics than does axiomatic set theory. Therefore a systematic philosophy of mathematics must begin as to subject matter with physics as expressed mathematically. Physics as a science is mathematical physics, so a philosophy of mathematics must be provided and some explanation given as to how and why empirical facts can be expressed mathematically. As the physical universe – the cosmos – is conceived as one reality existing in time and space without any individuality, a special problem arises in the philosophy of biology. Living beings are essential unities, organisms. Each living being and each human being is different from every other member of the same species. This character of individuality is completely absent from physical bodies, such as electrons, atoms, molecules, etc. The solution of this problem must wait until after the philosophy of mathematical physics is completed. This is no problem for an atheist or what I might call the logical atheist. For him, as there is no God, all reality is one of logical necessity – i.e. reality is a monism, there can be no essential difference between living beings and physical reality. All living organisms must be explained in purely physical terms. This must be, and of course is, the point of view of the atheist biologist Richard Dawkins.

The measurement of time

We now return to the consideration of the measurement of time, as this is the most fundamental of all measurement in physics. (The unit of distance, e.g. the metre, is not the most fundamental as it has been defined in terms of the distance travelled by light in a given time interval.) In the study of this problem I have the advantage of using the recent publication (1992) of the *Explanatory Supplement to the Astronomical Almanac*,[4] which has been completely revised and rewritten. The treatment of time is detailed and complicated, covering 48 pages and 128 references, but for our purpose a description of the different time scales and their relationship will be sufficient. There are four types or systems of time scale in common use:

1 Atomic time
2 Universal time, in which the unit of duration is based on the rotation of the earth
3 Sidereal time, in which the unit of duration is the period of the earth's rotation with respect to the stars
4 Dynamical time, based on the orbital motion of the earth, moon and planets

But this list of time scales is not based on the chronological order of the discovery and use of these scales. There is another list of time scales in the *Astronomical Almanac*, pages B4 and B5, which includes ephemeris time, in use from 1960 to 1983. The following is the list of time scales in their historical order of use:

1 Sidereal time
2 Universal time, or UT
3 Ephemeris time, or ET (1960–83)
4 Atomic time, or TAI (from 1972)
5 Dynamical time (from 1984)

Sidereal time is a measure of the rotation of the earth with respect to the stars. Universal time or UT is formally defined by a mathematical formula as a function of sidereal time. The sidereal day is four minutes shorter, i.e. 23 hours 56 minutes, than the mean solar day. It was always assumed that the rate of rotation of the celestial sphere was uniform, a belief that goes back to Aristotle in 350 BC. He believed that as the rotation was in a circle, which was the most perfect motion, it must be uniform. In recent times, with the development of very accurate clocks, the variation in the rate of rotation has been established. Even so, as recently as 1934 the best clocks then available could not show any variation in the rate of rotation. This is explained by Sir Harold Spencer Jones, the Astronomer Royal of the time:

It might be thought that clocks would provide a means of checking the period of rotation, but this is not possible, as the period is more constant than the rates of even the best clocks, so that the constancy of the period is used to check our clocks.[5]

But long before that date astronomers knew that there must be a variation in the rate of rotation of the earth. This is described in some detail in the new *Explanatory Supplement to the Astronomical Almanac*, Section 2.53: 'Rotation of the Earth'. There was a discrepancy between the observed and computed positions which revealed the difference between a measure of the earth's rotation and the measure of a uniform gravitational time. The discrepancies are most evident in the mean motion of the moon, due to the rapidity of its motion and the accuracy with which the inequalities can be observed. The variations in the earth's rotation (spin) also produce discrepancies in the observed motions of the bodies in the solar system in proportion to the magnitude of their respective mean motions. After a long series of studies by various astronomers, important papers by de Sitter (1927) and Spencer Jones, the Astronomer Royal (1939), correlated irregularities in the moon's motion with irregularities in the motion of the inner planets. The earth's rotation or spin was proved to be subject to variations. Since mean solar time was determined directly from sidereal observations, it could no longer be considered uniform. This was in effect a momentous conclusion. From the time of Aristotle it had been assumed – or in other words it was axiomatic – that the rate of rotation of the celestial sphere was uniform and gave the perfect measure of time. The great Copernican Revolution transferred the explanation of the rotation of the celestial sphere to the intrinsic spin of the earth. Now it was assumed or accepted as axiomatic that the rate of spin of the earth was uniform. However, astronomers subsequently proved that this rate of spin was not uniform. The accuracy of crystal-controlled clocks and later of atomic clocks confirmed the non-uniformity of the rate of spin of the earth. The time of celestial dynamics was now interpreted as the independent variable of the earth's orbital revolution around the sun. This independent variable was called ephemeris time or ET because it was based on the ephemerides, the predicted positions of the inner planets and the moon in their orbital motions around the sun and earth respectively. As described in detail in Section 2.55 – 'Ephemeris Time' – of the new *Explanatory Supplement* it was decided to redefine the fundamental unit of time – the second – as a fraction of the length of the year – the tropical year. After long discussions and conferences the final decision was made in 1960 at the 11th General Conference of Weights and Measures that the ephemeris was a fraction of the tropical year. The fraction was $\frac{1}{31,556,925.975}$ of the length of the tropical year for 1900 – i.e. 31.5 million seconds in the year (approximately). This is a momentous and fundamental change in the measurement of time, from the spin of the earth to the orbital motion of the earth around the sun according to the laws of celestial dynamics. The consequences of this most fundamental change in the measurement of time are more clearly and explicitly described in the first edition of the *Explanatory Supplement* of 1961:

> For astronomical purposes the most advantageous fundamental standard for the effective correlation and systematic representation of observed phenomena in terms of the measure of time is the independent variable of the accepted dynamical equations of motion. This measure of time may be characterised as the measure in which observed motions agree with the dynamical theories constructed from the laws of motion; in effect it is therefore defined by these laws.[6]

It goes on to say that this independent variable is 'uniform time'. It is assumed – in other words axiomatic – that the laws of motion expressed as equations are a perfect representation of the predicted positions of the planets and the moon.

Further refinement of the measurement of time was introduced in 1984. This was called dynamical time and replaced ephemeris time. But its basis was the same, namely the independent argument of dynamical time theories and ephemerides. These were of two scales of time, one of which – TDB – referred to the barycenter of the solar system, while the other was terrestrial dynamical time (TDT), taking into account factors involving the theory of relativity.

As the rate of spin of the earth is slowing down there is a difference between ET – ephemeris time and UT – universal time. The figures of the time scales are given on page K9 of the *Astronomical Almanac* each year. For 1983 the figures are:

    1960 – + 33.15
    1983 – + 52.96

This signifies for 23 years a difference of approximately 20 seconds – i.e. almost one second a year.

In 1971 the experimental atomic time scale was adopted as the world-wide time reference system under the name of international atomic time (TAI).

From January 1972 the difference between TAI and coordinated universal time (UTC) are listed on the same page K9 of the *Astronomical Almanac* – for the year 1993 they are:

    January 1972 + 10.00
    January 1991 + 26

This denotes, for a total of 19 years, a difference of 16 seconds, approximately one second per year. The difference between UTC and TAI is always an integral number of seconds. UTC is maintained in close agreement, to better than one second, with UT introducing extra seconds known as leap seconds to UTC, usually at the end of the last day of June or December. This lack of correspondence between the two scales of dynamical time and atomic time and universal time, each of which differs by approximately 1 second per year, indicates the rate of spin of the earth is slowing down 1 second in 31.5 million seconds. This might suggest a minute deviation from the conservation of angular momentum in the earth's rate of spin. The concept of dynamical time is based on time as the independent variable of the laws of motion as expressed by the equations of motion of celestial mechanics. If there is still any discrepancy in the predicted positions of the planets and the moon it can only be due to a lack of precision in the laws of motion themselves.

The Copernican Revolution

The most fundamental phenomenon of the natural world is the rotation of the celestial sphere. As we have been seen, it was the basis of the measurement of time and the alternation of night and day. Before the revolution in the Ptolemaic system of cosmology the earth was at the centre of the universe and at rest in two respects. It had no motion of translation, i.e. no motion from place to place, and no intrinsic spin. After the publication of Copernicus' *De Revolutionibus Orbium Coelestium* in the year of his death 1543, the sun was placed at the centre of the universe and the earth and the planets were in orbit around the sun. The earth also revolved on its axis and thereby accounted for the rotation of the celestial sphere. The earth now has two motions:

1   Translation – the orbital motion around the sun
2   Spin – intrinsic angulum momentum

The word 'rotation' is ambiguous. It can mean two different motions: the orbital motion, e.g. of the earth around the sun, which is a motion of translation from place to place, or the rotation of a body, again the earth, on its axis, i.e. spin. In spin the body remains in the same place and there is no translation – the motion is around the axis of spin. This word 'spin' is therefore unambiguous – it means intrinsic angular momentum. If the rotation of the celestial sphere is accepted as the most fundamental phenomenon of nature then it follows logically as a consequence of the Copernican Revolution that the spin of the earth is the most fundamental phenomenon of nature. All the planets and the moon are also the subject of spin, as well as the elementary particles of atomic physics, e.g. electrons. The motion of a body in translation is relative to some frame of reference. But the motion of spin does not require any frame of reference to describe it – the motion can be considered an absolute one. We now have the answer to the question: which of these motions, translation or spin, is the most fundamental and profound in the physical world? The answer is spin, not translatory motion. I am influenced in my conception of the importance of spin by Sir Edmund Whittaker's address on this subject as President of the Royal Society of Edinburgh in October 1944. The title of the address was 'Spin in the Universe'.[7] Whittaker describes spin as a universal phenomenon in nature: the earth and all the other members of the solar system rotate on their axes. He says that the motion of the earth's rotation on its axis can persist for a very long period of time. This is an example of the principle of conservation of spin or angular momentum, which states that spin remains permanently unaltered so long as there are no external forces. But it is rather surprising that Whittaker does not mention the evidence from the astronomers of his day that the rate of rotation or spin of the earth was not uniform, and could no longer be used as the perfect measure of time. He describes the discovery in 1925 that the electron has a spin, i.e. an intrinsic angular momentum. The amount of this spin must be a universal constant of nature. The final conclusion was that if Planck's constant of action divided by 2π is denoted by h (bar), then angular momentum or spin of the electron is $\tfrac{1}{2}h$ (bar); the photon or light corpuscle has the spin h (bar). Spin is a fundamental phenomenon of atomic theory or quantum mechanics. The spin of the earth and the other planets is also a most fundamental phenomenon of nature. This is why I maintain that spin is a more fundamental type of motion than the motion of translation, the movement of bodies from place to place. Later in his address Whittaker mentions the remarkable difference which exists, as regards relativity, between motions of rotation (meaning spin) and translation. In motions of translation we can only speak of the velocity of one body relative to another body, but Whittaker describes an optical experiment in 1925 which established that it was possible to deduce the angular velocity of the earth. Thus it is allowable to speak of velocities of rotation (spin) in an absolute manner, without the necessity of specifying any framework with respect to which the angular displacement takes place. The statement that some particular body is at rest as regards rotation (spin) is a statement that has meaning, although the statement that a particular body is at rest as regards translation, taken by itself, is meaningless. Whittaker concludes his address by observing that the explanation of spin in the universe is a still unsolved fundamental problem of cosmology.

The spin of the earth can be demonstrated visibly by Foucault's pendulum, first set up in Paris in 1851. Foucault also demonstrated the spin of the earth by the use of a gyroscope at about the same time. In 1993 I paid a special visit to see the Foucault's pendulum at the Science Museum in Kensington. It was set up by Sir Brian Pippard FRS in 1983, but is not very well publicised (I only found it by accident at the foot of one of the staircases) and is not mentioned in the leaflet given with the entrance ticket. I was disappointed that there is no demonstration of the earth's spin by means of a gyroscope, which would be more interesting and more dramatic as illustrating the most fundamental phenomenon of all nature. It is very remarkable that more than three hundred years had to pass from the Copernican Revolution of 1543 until 1851 when Foucault demonstrated visibly the spin of the earth with his pendulum. This could have been done at any time from 1543 by Galileo or any of the later astronomers, including Newton, yet none of them thought of doing so. It would have settled at once the controversy entailed by the Copernican Revolution. When Galileo uttered his famous words following his trial and condemnation by the Holy Office in Rome 1633 – *'Eppur si Muove'*, 'None the less it does move' – he meant of course the orbital motion of translation of the earth, not its revolution on its axis – its spin. Since the Copernican Revolution all or almost all the attention of astronomers has been focused on the orbital motion of the earth and the other planets and the moon. Newton's theory of gravitation is about this motion of translation around the sun. The same applies to Einstein's theory of relativity: both the special theory and the general theory of gravitation are concerned with the motion of translation of objects and all the planets and the moon. However, the motion of translation is relative to some frame of reference, i.e. to another body or place, as is shown by the very name of Einstein's theory – the theory of *relativity*. The motion of spin, on the other hand, is not a relative one – it is absolute, no frame of reference is required. This was pointed out by Whittaker, as has already been described. In the pre-Copernican cosmology the rotation of the celestial sphere was assumed to be uniform – i.e. it was axiomatic. After the Copernican Revolution, this rotation or spin was transferred to the earth and the concept of the uniformity of that spin was retained. This uniformity of spin was the basis of the measurement of time until it was proved that the spin of the earth was not uniform, as we saw earlier. This made necessary the change of the measure of time, from one based on the spin of the earth to one based on its orbital motion around the sun. The latter was the basis of ephemeris time, which was introduced in 1960, and the further refinement furnished by the introduction of dynamical time in 1984.

There is a very important phenomenon in astronomy – precession – which is related to the spin of the earth. The celestial pole which is in the direction of the axis of rotation or spin of the earth is not fixed in space. It moves in a circle because of gravitation forces (mainly from the moon and sun) acting on the earth. The period of general or lunisolar precession is about 26,000 years. This was discovered by the Greek astronomer Hipparchus in about 150 BC and was called the precession of the equinoxes, since it results in the slow westward motion of the equinoxes about the ecliptic.

It is only in recent years that an intensive study has been made of the phenomenon of the rotation, or spin, of the earth. This is described in some detail in Chapter 4, Section 4 of the new *Explanatory Supplement to the Astronomical Almanac* (1992), with the title 'The Monitoring of the Rotation of the Earth'. The word 'rotation' means of course rotation on its axis – the spin. Several very special methods are being used for this monitoring, e.g. Lunar Laser-Ranging (LLR), Satellite Laser-Ranging (SLR) and Very Long

Baseline Interferometry (VLBI). A more exotic method for determining variations in the earth's rotation is the use of Laser-Ring Gyroscopes. On 1 January 1988 the International Earth Rotation Service (IERS) began operations under the auspices of the International Astronomical Union. The title of the former body indicates the very special scientific studies now being made of the spin of the earth and its variation. A most important function of the IERS is given in the following quotation:

> The I.E.R.S. is also responsible for deciding when a step in U.T.C. is necessary in order to keep it within 0.75 of U.T.I. These steps, commonly known as *Leap seconds*, may be positive or negative, are of 1 second duration, are announced at least 8 weeks ahead of time, and may be inserted at the end of any month (preferably in practice at the end of June or December). Since their introduction in 1972, these steps have always been positive and have been required every six months to 2 years. A table of these steps is given in the current Astronomical Almanac, p K9 as differences U.T.C. from T.A.I.[8]

I do not understand why it is stated that the steps may be positive or negative when in reality all the steps have been positive, as shown quite clearly on page K9 of the *Astronomical Almanac*. These have already been given earlier and show an increasing difference between TAI – atomic time – and UTC – universal time – of 1 second per year, i.e. the rate of spin of the earth is slowing down 1 second in one year of 31.5 million seconds. I was disappointed that the table of differences was not printed in the *Almanac*. If there is a departure from the uniformity of spin of the earth which is regular it might indicate some fundamental natural phenomenon which might possibly be a deviation from the conservation of intrinsic angular momentum.

The phenomenon of spin

It would be useful to list the various factors associated with the phenomenon of spin:

1   The rate of spin can be uniform or non-uniform. The rate is given as revolutions per second, and expressed as radians per second.

2   A spinning body has one axis which can have three and only three directions in space. The three directions are:
   a)   north – positive +
        south – negative –
   b)   east – positive +
        west – negative –
   c)   up – positive +
        down – negative –

These three directions can be expressed as vectors with signs + or − as indicated.

3   No coordinates are required: spin is coordinate-free.

4   Spin is motion − therefore the factor of time is required. The number expressing time is a scalar number.

5   The motion of spin is absolute not relative.

6   The motion of spin has two and only two directions − left-handed and right-handed.

7   Spin is associated with the phenomenon of precession. When a torque is applied to the axis of spin − e.g. of a gyroscope − it turns about an axis at right angles to:
    a)   the axis to which torque was applied
    b)   the main axis of spin.

Things subject to spin include tops, gyroscopes, the earth and all the other planets, and also atomic particles, e.g. electrons and photons. Therefore spin is a universal phenomenon as stated by Sir Edmund Whittaker. It is to be contrasted with the motion of a body from place to place, i.e. the motion of translation. A body can move from place to place on a plane − which requires only two dimensions. But translatory motion can also be in three dimensions, such as on a spiral staircase or a spiral ramp − this is motion in a helix.

The motion of spin always requires three dimensions of space for its description because the axis of spin can be in the three different directions of space − phenomenological space, i.e. the space of human experience. This is the space of stereoscopic vision, in which objects appear to have solidity and to have not two dimensions but three. The word is from the Greek *stereos*, meaning 'solid'. The same concept applies to the differences in the relative positions in space (of three dimensions) of the atoms in a molecule. If the atoms in the molecule are non-symmetrical, it is possible to have two forms of the molecule, one the mirror image of the other. The solutions of these chemicals can differ by one of the two forms rotating the plane of polarised light to the right and the other − the mirror image − rotating the light to the left. There is no doubt that the motion of spin in nature is more fundamental than motion from place to place, i.e. translatory motion. The word 'rotation', as already mentioned, is ambiguous; its two meanings refer to two different states of affairs. In the first, a body, e.g. a planet, can rotate in an orbit in translation from place to place. The other meaning is of the body rotating on its axis − or spin. The motion of translation can have any number of different directions, but the motion of spin has the unique property of having two and only two directions: right-handed (clockwise) and left-handed (anticlockwise). The atomic physicists use the language of spin-up (left-handed) and spin-down (right-handed). (This language cannot be used for a gyroscope with spin in the other two directions of three-dimensional space, namely east and west, and north and south.) Since all phenomena of nature must be expressed mathematically, there is no science of physics without mathematics; thus all physics is mathematical physics. We now have to ask the question: what is the mathematics of the most fundamental phenomenon, spin? The answer is Hamilton's quaternions. These have already been described in the section on quaternions in Chapter 3, where I concluded that the symbols $i, j,$ k represented the three axes of spin:

$$ij = +k$$
$$ji = -k$$

This signified the reversal of the order of multiplication of i and j, i.e. the noncommutative multiplication of i and j resulted in the change of the third vector k from + to –, i.e. reversing its direction and in consequence reversing the direction of spin. The vector k is then at right angles to i and j. But there was some lingering doubt whether my interpretation was correct. I remembered reading Hamilton's description and explanation of quaternions as given to Lady Rosse during a visit to the great Birr telescope in 1848. This is given in Sean O'Donnell's biography of Hamilton.[9] To assist him in his explanation, Hamilton used a penknife held horizontally. The handle was called i and the blade j. The operation ij resulted in the *blade* being *upwards* and the operation ji resulted in the *handle* being *downwards*. The result of these operations on the same pair of vectors which the handle and blade represent, was that the vector upwards and the vector downwards were different. I found this difficult to follow and it is doubtful if Lady Rosse was able to understand it either. On reading the account again I was very relieved to find that the paradoxical formula which Hamilton was explaining was $ij = -ji$, and not $ij = ji$. In using the blade and handle of the penknife Hamilton is assuming two different vectors for his explanation, and of course the penknife is completely static and has nothing to do with spin and the axis of spin. If i, j, k are the axes of spin only one axis is required, which can be in the three directions of space:

$+i$ – east; $-i$ – west
$+j$ – north; $-j$ – south
$+k$ – upwards; $-k$ – downwards

The standard formulas for the quaternion symbols i, j, k, are:

$$i^2 = j^2 = k^2 = i\,j\,k = -1$$
$$ij = -ji = k$$
$$jk = -kj = i$$
$$ki = -ik = j$$

110

But Hamilton gives the symbols in a different form in his communication of November 1843,[10] and gives them again in the same form in Section 60 of the preface to his *Lectures on Quaternions*.[11] These are set out in three columns as follows:

$i^2 = -1$	$j^2 = -1$	$k^2 = -1$	A
$ij = +k$	$jk = +i$	$ki = +j$	B
$ji = -k$	$kj = -i$	$ik = -j$	C

The symbols i, j, k are all imaginary. Each is equal to $\sqrt{-1}$, so their squares are equal to -1. The non-commutative multiplication in each of the three columns results in a third vector which has two different directions represented by $+$ and -1. It is quite obvious from these formulas that $ij + ji = 0$; $jk + kj = 0$; $ki + ik = 0$. Professor A.W. Conway FRS mentions in a paper on Hamilton's life and work that he took the tremendous step of making $ij + ji = 0$. The above formulation of the symbols in the three columns A, B and C makes it easy to see how that was possible.

Now, using the concept that i, j, k represent the three axes of spin in Euclidean space, the symbols are vectors and $+$ and $-$ represent opposite directions of spin:

$+i$ = east; $+j$ = north; $+k$ = up
$-i$ = west; $-j$ = south; $-k$ = down

By applying spin to each vector or axis – of which there are only two directions, left and right – we have:

$+i$ = left spin	$+j$ = right spin	$+k$ = left spin
$-i$ = right spin	$-j$ = left spin	$-k$ = right spin

$ij = +k$ = left spin – spin up
$ji = -k$ = right spin – spin down

$jk = +i$ = left spin
$kj = -i$ = right spin

$ki = +j$ = right spin
$ik = -j$ = left spin

In each case the multiplication of the pair of symbols which are vectors results in a third vector which is at right angles to each of the original pair. Changing the order of multiplication results in the third vector – the same vector – reversing its direction and in consequence reversing the direction of spin. The quaternions can be demonstrated by using a knitting needle through an apple, which represents the single axis of spin. Reversing the needle will result in the reversal of the direction of spin. But if this was demonstrated before a class of bright children I would be surprised if one of them did not say 'But sir, the apple is not spinning.' He or she would be perfectly correct. The complete demonstration should be with a gyroscope spinning at high speed. Better still to use a pair of gyroscopes, one with right-hand spin and the other with left-hand spin. The phenomenon of precession seems to be represented in each of the formulas, e.g. in the formula $ij = +k$, ij represents a torque applied to the one axis of spin, resulting in the motion or precession of the axis to a third position $+k$ (up) at right angles to i and j. If the spin was in the opposite direction the motion or precession would be in the opposite direction, i.e. $-k$ (down). The symbols i, j, k are only three in number, but 'quaternion' means four numbers. Hamilton for a time thought of using a different name – *grammarithm*, from the Greek words for line and number. The line was a directed line, i.e. a vector and the number was a scalar number. The full formula for a quaternion can be given in the following symbolism:

$$q = w + ix + jy + kz$$

Here, w, x, y, z, the last four letters of the alphabet, are all scalar numbers. The first letter remains separate, the last three letters are each coupled with i, j, k, which represent the length of each vector, or in the case of spin, the rate of spin. The letter w represents the scalar number or part, while $ix + jy + kz$ represent the vector part.

Using the first four letters of the alphabet the quaternion is:

$$q = a + ib + jc + kd$$
$$a = \text{scalar part}$$
$$ib + jc + kd = \text{vector part}$$

However, the letters coupling with i, j, k are now b, c, d, the second, third and fourth letters of the alphabet, which loses the symmetry of the symbolism. If d is 0 the latter formulation leaves us with $a + ib + jc$, which is Hamilton's triplet which he had such great difficulty in multiplying. This can also be written as $a + bi + cj$. This is an alternative convention in the coupling of the scalar numbers with i, j, k. The symbolism looks better with i, j, k before each scalar number and that will be used consistently. If c is 0 in the formula we are left with $a + ib$, which is the complex number. If b, c and d are all 0 we are left with the pure scalar number a. There is a simple and useful solution to the problem of using the first three letters or the last three letters of the alphabet to couple with i, j, k. The solution is to use the initial letter s to represent the scalar part of the quaternion. Therefore $s = \text{scalar}$. The formula for the quaternion then is:

$q = s + ia + jb + kc$ – i.e. using the first three letters
$q = s + ix + jy + kz$ – i.e. using the last three letters

By this means the symmetry of the symbolism is maintained. The symbol s in each case is the scalar part of the quaternion. The vector part is $ia + jb + kc$ and $ix + jy + kz$. The quaternion is the sum of a scalar and vector part:

$$q = s + v$$

The vector part of the quaternion has three different vectors representing the three different directions in three-dimensional Euclidean space. With the concept of i, j, k representing the axis of spin, the three different directions which the one axis of spin can have in tridimensional space are east–west, north–south and up–down. There are only three dimensions in space – phenomenological space, the space of human experience. There are not four dimensions of space, only three.

As already stated, the quaternion as the sum of a scalar and vector part suggested to Hamilton the name *grammarithm*, meaning a line – a directed line, a vector – and a number – a scalar number. But the name does not quite fit the symbolism $q = s + v$, as the number is first and the line – the vector – is second – the opposite of the exact derivation of the word. To fit the name exactly the equation should be $q = v + s$; i.e. with the vector first and the number – the scalar – second.

Sean O'Donnell in his biography of Hamilton gives a quotation from Cornelius Lanczos, of which the last sentence is 'Today we are to call d the "time part" and ai + bj + ck the "space part" of the quaternion q.' When I first read that I had difficulty in understanding it, I did not know where the d came from. On reading Lanczos's article, of which I have a photocopy, the explanation was very simple. The formula which he gave for a quaternion is:

$$q = ai + bj + ck + d$$

He has reversed the usual symbolism for a quaternion, putting the scalar part at the end instead of at the beginning, i.e. $q = v + s$. The reason for doing that seems to be to use the first three letters of the alphabet to couple with i, j, k. It is confusing to have such different symbolisms for the quaternion. The solution of this problem as already given is to use a separate symbol – s – for the scalar part of the quaternion:

$$q = s + ia + jb + kc$$

This is the symbolism used by Professor Don M. Yost in his excellent article on quaternions in the *McGraw-Hill Encyclopaedia of Science and Technology* (7th edn,) 1992, in which s is the 'time-part' – the scalar part –

and $ia + jb + kc$ is the 'space part' or vector part of the quaternion q. Lanczos's formula has the merit of matching exactly Hamilton's term *grammarithm* because the line – the vector – is first and the number – the scalar – second. The problem of the meaning of the scalar part of the quaternion will be investigated later. Hamilton had the greatest difficulty in trying to decide what was its meaning and what it could represent in reality.

The well-known fact that Hamilton discovered quaternions in a sudden flash of inspiration on 16 October 1843 obscures the fact that he spent more than ten years of constant effort in trying to work out their solution. The fact that the greatest mathematician of the nineteenth century took so long to discover them is an indication of the greatest difficulty of the problem. The task before Hamilton seemed clear enough: complex numbers of form $a + ib$ were taken as representing vectors in the plane, i.e. two dimensions, of space. The problem was to extend the number system to vectors in the three dimensions of space. The complex numbers could be called double algebra for two units, so by analogy Hamilton should have required triple algebra or triplets for the three dimensions of space.

The properties that Hamilton hoped his new numbers would have are given in a list of six as described by Michael Crowe in an excellent work *A History of Vector Analysis*. They are briefly as follows:

1   The associative property for addition and multiplication
2   The commutative property for addition and multiplication
3   The distributive property
4   The property that division is unambiguous
5   The law of the moduli
6   The property that the new numbers would have a significant interpretation in terms of three-dimensional space.[12]

Hamilton was able to preserve all of the properties 1–5 of the operation in algebra as above, except that the multiplication was non-commutative. The sixth property listed, that the new numbers – the quaternions – should have a significant or meaningful interpretation in three dimensions of space, is open to different opinions. My interpretation is that the symbols i, j, k represent the three directions in space of the one axis of a body subject to spin. The most detailed account of the various steps taken by Hamilton in the solution of his problem is given by B.L. Van der Waerden in his article 'Hamilton's Discovery of Quaternions'.[13] The subtitle of the article refers to Hamilton's repeated failures until the final leap into the fourth dimension. I will not go into all the steps taken by Hamilton but will concentrate attention on the crucial one – called by Van der Waerden 'the leap into the fourth dimension'. Hamilton began with his triplets $a + bi + cj$ or $a + ib + jc$. In the formula a is a scalar number, ib and jc are vectors. Van der Waerden quotes Hamilton's letter to Graves on 17 October 1843: 'and here there dawned on me the notion that we must admit in some sense a fourth dimension of space for the purpose of calculating with triplets'. This fourth dimension appeared as a 'paradox' to Hamilton himself and he hastened to transfer the paradox to algebra. The letter continues:

> . . . or transferring the paradox to algebra [we] must admit a *third* distinct imaginary symbol k, not to be confused with either i or j, but equal to the product of the first as multiplier and the second as multiplied; and therefore I was led to introduce *quaternions* such as a + ib + jc + kd or a b c d.[14]

In the above formula *a* is a scalar number – i.e. the scalar part of the quaternion – while *ib + jc + kd* is the vector part, totally different from the scalar part. Van der Waerden goes on to mention multidimensional geometry and Cayley's geometry of *n*-dimensions. But Hamilton is only concerned to devise a number system from the two dimensions of complex numbers to the three dimensions of the space of the natural real world. Van der Waerden then continues (p. 231): 'after Hamilton had introduced ij = –ji = k as a fourth independent basis vector, he continued the calculation . . .'

But stating *k* as a fourth independent vector is contradicting what Hamilton has said. Van der Waerden has correctly quoted Hamilton as above: 'we must admit a *third* distinct imaginary symbol k'. Therefore the correct account is *k* is the third vector, not the fourth. Hamilton then realised that $k^2 = -1$ is necessary to fulfil the law of the moduli. He then said that his assumptions were now completed:

$$i^2 = j^2 = k^2 = -1$$

The quaternion or set of four numbers is therefore:

$$q = a + ib + jc + kd$$

Here, *a* is the scalar part of the quaternion, *ib + jc + kd* is the vector part, and *i, j, k* are the three vectors of the real or phenomenological world of three dimensions, which is what Hamilton was aiming for. The problem now is what is the meaning of the first number represented by *a*? It is not another dimension of space but a scalar number, unidimensional and extending from + ∞ to –∞. Van der Waerden does not mention in his article that a quaternion has two parts, the scalar plus a vector part. Hamilton later changed his mind about the possibilities of a fourth dimension and came to the conclusion that *a* – the scalar part – represented time. In a paper communicated to the Royal Irish Academy in November 1844 he referred to the scalar aspect or number in quaternions:

> and the progression on this scale from negative to positive infinity, obtained by

combining a quantitative element with the contrast between two opposite directions, corresponds less to the conception of space itself (though we have seen that considerations of space might have suggested it) than to the conception of *time;* the variety which it admits is not tri- but uni-dimensional; and it would, in the language of some philosophical systems, be said to appertain rather to the notion of *intensive* than of extensive magnitude.[15]

The problem is again referred to by Hamilton in Section 60 of his preface to *Lectures on Quaternions*, in which he mentions 'a product being here regarded as a FOURTH PROPORTIONAL, to a certain *Extra-spatial unit*, and to two directed factors – lines in space'. The word 'Extra-spatial' has a footnote:

It seemed (and still seems) to me natural to connect this *Extra-spatial unit* with the conception [3] of TIME, regarded here merely as an axis of continuous and uni-dimensional progression.[16]

The number 3 as used in this footnote refers to Section 3 of the preface of Hamilton's essay of 1835, in which he considered algebra as both the science of order in progression and the science of pure time. At the end of Section 60 of the preface Hamilton makes a very important statement about quaternions – a quaternion is considered as the quotient of two directed lines in tridimensional space. It is quite clear from that definition that Hamilton considered quaternions as describing three-dimensional space and not four-dimensional space.

In the next section of the preface, Section 61, at the mention of multiplication in algebra, Hamilton has a footnote about Professor H. Grassmann's work, the *Ausdehnungslehre*, published at Leipzig in 1844. He states that he did not read it until years after the invention of his quaternions. Grassmann states in the preface to his work that he had not succeeded in extending the use of imaginaries from the plane to space. The 'space' meant here is of course the space of three dimensions. This is exactly what Hamilton had achieved in his calculus of quaternions.

The whole system of the quaternions is so comprehensive and complicated that it can have different interpretations and uses. There is the algebraic aspect and the geometrical interpretation, which Hamilton also developed as well as the algebraic. P.G. Tait, Hamilton's principal disciple and promoter of quaternions, particularly stresses the geometrical form of the quaternions in his book *An Elementary Treatise on Quaternions*[17] (1867). He mentions in the preface to that work that the algebraic interpretation may be interesting to the pure analyst but it is repulsive to the student of physics, who should consider *i*, *j*, *k* from the first as geometrical realities – not as algebraic imaginaries. 'Repulsive' is very strong language to use. Tait thought that the geometrical interpretation was more useful in applications to physics, but it is quite clear that these applications to physics did not include spin. Tait said that the ratio of two vectors or the multiplier required to change one vector into another depends on four numbers – a quaternion. Hamilton's concept was the same, as shown by his use of the penknife to explain quaternions: the blade and the handle are two vectors, and there is no suggestion of the motion of spin – the model used is completely static.

With the concept of spin, quaternions can have a different interpretation or meaning. Bodies which are the subject of spin – e.g. tops, gyroscopes and the earth – have one axis of spin only. That one axis of spin can be in the three directions of tridimensional space of the natural real world – north–south, east–west and up–down – and of course in all intermediate positions or angles. These three directions are represented by i, j, k. I should mention at this point that in the quaternions i represented the directions east and west, but in complex numbers the real axis x is east–west and the imaginary axis y is north–south represented by i. It seems strange that the representation of the symbols was changed – i in quaternions should be north–south and j east–west to keep the extension of the symbols from complex numbers to quaternions the same.

The motion of spin is absolute, not relative as it is with the motion of a body in translation from place to place. Since all motion including spin is in time, a number is required to represent time. This is the first number of the set of four numbers of the quaternion – $q = a + ib + jc + kd$ – i.e. the scalar number. (Lanczos's version of the quaternion formula, as described earlier in this chapter, is rather confusing in that it simply has d as the final part of the formula.) Using the symbol s for scalar, the quaternion is:

$$q = s + ia + jb + kc \quad \text{using the first three letters of the alphabet}$$
$$\text{or} \quad q = s + ix + jy + kz \quad \text{using the last three letters of the alphabet}$$

This clearly and explicitly indicates the two parts of the quaternion – the scalar and vector parts.

Time is s – the scalar element – which Hamilton conceded as extending from $+ \infty$ to $- \infty$, i.e. time with no beginning, extending to infinity in the past. But if time had a beginning the scale would begin at 0; that would be an absolute scale of time, just like the Kelvin scale of temperature. This time with a beginning would be asymmetric, it would have an arrow; forward and backward would be different. It is the unique character of spin to have two and only two directions – right-handed and left-handed. If the spin is uniform, then right-handed and left-handed are equal – the equation of motion of spin is commutative. If there is a change in the rate of spin, left-hand and right-hand spin are not equal – the equation of motion for that changing rate of spin would be non-commutative or, more properly, anti-commuting. As time with a beginning has a direction, i.e. it can be conceived as a vector or (as Hamilton called it) a step in time. – e.g. from 1920 to 1930 – then steps, intervals or duration in time are vectors. Then the quaternion would have four vectors –

one for time and three for space – i.e. not four vectors for space, only three. Space and time are completely different in concept: there is no leap into the fourth dimension. The vectors i, j, k representing the one axis of spin can rotate into the three directions of space and all intermediate directions, but time, being unidimensional, has two and only two directions – forward and backward. The three directions of space are all equal, but the two directions of time – forward and backward – are not equal, especially if time has the character of being asymmetric. The importance and special value of the concept that quaternions are the mathematics of spin seems to me to be related to the unique fact that spin has two and only two directions, right-handed and left-handed. It is evident that there is an analogy or, more correctly, a correlation between the two directions of spin and the two directions of time. The interpretation of the quaternion formula $ij = +k$ and $ji = -k$ therefore is that the operation of the multiplication ij results in the third vector k being in the direction upwards – i.e. left-handed spin. The multiplication ji – i.e. with the order reversed – results in the same vector k being downward – i.e. right-handed spin. The reversal of the order of multiplication of i and j results in the reversal of the direction of the third vector k and obviously in consequence the reversal of the direction of spin. For this whole process to take place three dimensions of space are required. This would be impossible if space had four, five, six or ten dimensions of space. How could a gyroscope spin in ten dimensions of space?

The natural, the real world, the world of experience – i.e. the phenomeno-logical world – in which we human beings live has three dimensions and only three and that is sufficient to explain the most important phenomenon of spin. It is useful to give some account of how I came to the concept of quaternions as the mathematics of spin as given in the following list:

1   The influence of Sir Edmund Whittaker's address to the Royal Society of Edinburgh on 'Spin in the Universe'.
2   Whittaker's comments on the possible rehabilitation of quaternions for quantum theory – his statement that the spin-matrices introduced by Pauli in 1927 are Hamilton's three quaternion units i, j, k.
3   George Temple's book *100 Years of Mathematics* (1981). In it he mentions the usefulness of quaternions in the theory of tops and gyro-scopes. The latter are the perfect models of spin.
4   The interest for many years in the rotation (spin) of the earth in the measurement of time, the discovery of the non-uniformity of the rate of spin and the introduction of ephemeris time in consequence.
5. Reading Sean O'Donnell's account of the commutative law and non-commutative multiplication in his biography of Hamilton (1983). In such mathematics the order of multiplication makes a difference – and multiplication is equivalent to rotation. Hamilton explained that:

$ij = +k$ (the vector upwards)
$ji = -k$ (the same vector downwards)

If $+k$ is the axis of spin and it is left-handed, then $-k$ is the same axis of spin but right-handed. The non-commutative multiplication reverses the same axis of spin and in consequence changes or reverses its direction from left-handed spin to right-handed spin. I did not obtain this idea from Hamilton or Tait because it is not present in the writings of these two eminent philosophers of mathematics.

In trying to understand quaternions I cut three pieces of cardboard shaped like arrows to represent the three vectors i, j, k, but without any success. Then I remembered Hamilton's explanation of quaternions for Lady Rosse as described earlier – the blade and the handle of the penknife are *two* vectors. Finally I put a knitting needle through the centre of an apple to represent the axis of spin. Only one axis is required: that is the secret of the successful understanding of spin. There is only one axis, which can be in the three different directions north–south, east–west and up–down and in all inter-mediate positions or angles. These were the quaternions units i, j, k. It was immediately obvious that if you reverse the single axis of spin, you reverse the direction of spin. For the complete demonstration you should have a gyroscope which is spinning or better still a pair of gyroscopes, one with right-hand spin and the other with left-hand spin. The axis of the spinning gyroscope is in the three dimensions of the space of Euclidean geometry.

The next problem is to consider the development of vector analysis by Gibbs and others and how it differs from Hamilton's quaternions.

7 Quaternions versus vector analysis

The study of vector analysis is greatly facilitated by Michael Crowe's book *A History of Vector Analysis*, which charts the evolution of the idea of a vectorial system. This most important and valuable work was first published in 1967 by the University of Notre Dame Press, and a new edition by Dover was published in 1985. The latter had a new preface with numerous references to more recent publications; these included Volume 3 of Hamilton's *Mathematical Papers* (1967) and the biographies of Hamilton by Thomas Hankins (1980) and by Sean O'Donnell (1983). The notes to the preface contain full references to all the recent publications. There was a new Dover edition of the book in 1994, containing a publisher's note stating that the exceptional merits of the book were recognised by it being awarded, in an international competition in 1992, a Jean Scott prize of $4000 by the Maison des Sciences de L'Homme in Paris. In the preface to the first edition of 1967 Michael Crowe makes the following important comment:

> Despite the importance of Vector analysis its history has been little studied. Not a single book and not more than a handful of scholarly papers have up to now been written on its history. Consequently many historical errors may be found in the relevant literature.[1]

It is a most remarkable fact that Crowe's book of 1967 is the first adequate study of vector analysis, considering the importance of the latter for mathematics and mathematical physics.

A special feature of the book is the great number of references to the mathematical literature at the end of each chapter. These are of great value for further study and research in the field of vector analysis.

To begin my study of the relationship between quaternions and vector analysis I propose to use the excellent article by Reginald J. Stephenson on 'Development of Vector Analysis from Quaternions' published in 1966. The article as a whole can be summed up by the long paragraph at its beginning:

> About the middle of the last century, there were invented several forms of multiple algebra, some of which are extensively used today in mathematical physics. The two types discussed here are quaternions, a quadruple algebra, and vector analysis, a triple algebra. The notations and forms of analysis, used in the two systems are contrasted using for each their presentation of scalar and vector products and of Gauss's, Stoke's and Green's theorems. Maxwell made use of the vector part of quaternions in his treatise on Electricity and it was largely due to this that Gibbs came to invent his form of vector analysis. By 1890, about fifty years after the invention of quaternions, it became apparent that Gibbs's vector analysis was being used in place of quaternions, and this gave rise to a heated controversy in the pages of *Nature*. In the seventy years since this controversy, it is apparent that Gibbs's work and point of view have been completely vindicated.[2]

The simplest way to change from quaternions – a set of four numbers, i.e. quadruple algebra – to vector analysis – a set of three numbers, i.e. triple algebra – is to remove one of the numbers. The quaternions formula can be written using either the first four letters of the alphabet or the last four letters:

$a + ib + jc + kd$
or
$w + ix + jy + kz$

Here, a, b, c, d and w, x, y, z are all scalar numbers, while i, j, k are vectors whose squares are -1:

$i^2 = j^2 = k^2 = -1$

To keep the symmetry of the symbols we can use the first three letters of the alphabet and the last three letters of the alphabet to couple with i, j, and k and use s (for 'scalar') for the first symbol:

$s + ia + jb + kc$
$s + ix + jy + kz$

If, in the formula using the first four letters of the alphabet ($a + ib + jc + kd$), you remove the last part (kd), you are left with $a + ib + jc$ – this was the formula for the triplets which Hamilton was thinking about for more than ten years but without any success in their multiplication. He could add and subtract them but failed to multiply them until he realised that the multiplication must be non-commutative. If c and d in the first formula are negative you are left with $a + ib$, which is the complex number. If b, c and d are all negative you are left with a, which is the scalar number – a real number. This neatly shows that quaternions are an extension of complex numbers.

Hamilton's final opinion was that the first symbol a or w – i.e. the scalar number – represented time. It is useful to represent this by s – obviously for scalar, not space. For vector analysis it is the first symbol a, w or s which is removed: this is the time part of the quaternion, leaving the last three symbols – $ib + jc + kd$ or $ix + ij + kz$ – which are the vector part or space part of the quaternion. Hamilton explains so clearly and beautifully the scalar part and vector part of the quaternion that it must be given in his own words, as taken from Volume 3, Chapter 2, Part VIII, Section 18 of his *Mathematical Papers*:

> The operation of the Real and imaginary parts of a quaternion is an operation of such frequent occurrence, and may be regarded as being so fundamental in this theory, that it is convenient to introduce symbols which shall denote concisely the two separate results of this operation. The algebraically *Real* part may receive, according to the question in which it occurs, all values contained on the one *scale* of progression of number from negative to positive infinity; we shall call it therefore the *scalar* part or simply the *scalar* of the quaternion, and shall form its symbol by prefixing, to the symbol of the quaternion, the characteristic scal., or simply S., where no confusion seems likely to arise from using this last abbreviation. On the other hand, the algebraically imaginary part, being geo-metrically constructed by a straight line or Radius vector, which has in general, for each determined quaternion, a determined length and determined direction in space, may be called the *vector part* or simply the *vector* of the quaternion; and may be denoted by prefixing the characteristic vect or V. We may therefore say that a quaternion is in general the sum of its own scalar and vector parts and may be write
>
> $Q = $ Scal. $Q + $ Vect $Q = $ S.$Q + $ V.Q
> or simply – $Q = $ S.$Q + $ V.Q[3]

The quaternion then has two parts: the scalar or real part and the vector part, the imaginary or space part. The scalar part represents time.

The quaternion has four units, the first the real or scalar part and the other three the vector part or space part which are all imaginary:

Four quaternion units

Time	Space
1 scalar	3 vectors
Real	All imaginary

Hamilton mentions in the preface to his *Lectures on Quaternions* that he had considered another name for quaternions, i.e. 'GRAMMARITHM from the two Greek words *gramme*, a line and *arithmos* a number'.[4]

The line of course is the vector part and the number the scalar part. This can be represented in a very simple diagram in which the number – x – represents the scalar part and the line the vector part:

Vector 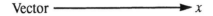 x

But that does not correctly represent the standard quaternion formula $s + v$, in which the scalar or real number comes first and the vector part is next. In the word 'grammarithm', the vector part – the line – is first and the number part second. The correct expression should be 'arithmogramm', i.e. with the number first and the line or vector next, e.g.

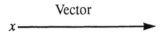

The Hungarian mathematician Cornelius Lanczos had special knowledge and appreciation of Hamilton and his quaternions. Lanczos, who is briefly mentioned as a collaborator of Einstein in Abraham Pais' biography of Einstein, gave a public lecture in commemoration of the hundredth anniversary of Hamilton's death (2 September 1865). He gives an interesting account of Hamilton's discovery of quaternions:

> Two imaginary units were not enough, three were in fact needed: i, j, k. These three units had to play a completely symmetrical role, to take cognisance of the fact that there are no preferential directions in space, one axis being just as good as any other axis. Hence the number triplet had to appear in the form ai + bj + ck; but to this an ordinary number d has to be added, so that a full fledged quaternion (this name was already settled in his mind, when he arrived at the academy) must appear in the form
>
> q = ai + bj + ck + d.
>
> It was not enough to operate with a three dimensional world, one had to go into a world of *four* dimensions, in which the position of a point is characterised by *four* numbers; a, b, c, d.[5]

Lanczos called *d* the time part and *ai + bj + ck* the space part of the quaternion. But this is a complete change of order of the symbols of the quaternion. Hamilton's triplets cannot now be derived from the formula and the symbols for the complex number have disappeared. The time part of the quaternion is deliberately changed from the first number or place to the fourth place. This is a complete reversal of the standard formula for quaternions as used by Hamilton. But it does fit the name 'grammarithm', which Hamilton thought of using. The line – the vector or space point – is first, while the number – the scalar part, the real number – is second.

Lanczos mentions going into a world of four dimensions, but the spatial world has only three dimensions. By analogy with space, time can be called a fourth dimension. But other language and concepts for the four sets of numbers of the quaternion can be used. The mathematician L.E. Dickson in his paper 'On Quaternions and Their Generalization and the History of the Eight Square Theorem' does not use the language of dimensions:

> We have now accomplished one of the aims of the paper, having exhibited linear algebras in 2, 4, 8 units for which the norm of a product equals the product of the norms of the factors (thus giving the 2, 4, and 8 square theorems) and such that, if the coordinates of the numbers of the algebra be restricted to be real numbers, both right-handed and left-handed division except by zero are possible and unique.
>
> While the three algebras have in common these two fundamental properties, they differ in other respects. For complex numbers multiplication is both commutative and associative, for quaternions it is associative but not commutative, for Cayley's algebra of 8 units it is neither commutative nor associative.[6]

The algebra in two units are complex numbers; the algebra in four units are quaternions. Three of the units are referring to space – they can be dimensions of space in the three directions east–west, north–south and up and down and in all intermediate directions. The first unit of the quaternions – the scalar part – represents time which has two directions and only two directions, forward and backward. The scalar number for time is a real number whose square is positive. The three numbers for space i, j, k are all imaginary; their squares are equal to -1.

Josiah Willard Gibbs

The American mathematician Gibbs (1839–1903) created modern vector analysis. In 1879 he gave a course in vector analysis, and in 1881 he arranged for the private printing of the first half of his *Elements of Vector Analysis*, with the second half following in 1884. These papers were not published but were circulated privately to leading mathematicians and physicists. It was only in 1901 that the first formally published book entirely devoted to presenting the modern system of vector analysis appeared. This was Edwin Bidwell Wilson's book *Vector Analysis: A Text Book for the Use of Students of Mathematics and Physics Founded upon the Lectures of J. Willard Gibbs*. It is rather remarkable that it took so long for such a work to be published. Michael Crowe in his *History of Vector Analysis*, first published in 1967, gives a detailed account of that history. Hamilton was the first to use the concept of the vector – a real number with direction in space. This was the vector part of his quaternions, which he discovered in 1843. His *Lectures on Quaternions* were published in 1853, and his *Elements of Quaternions* in 1866, the year after his death. Peter Guthrie Tait, Hamilton's principal disciple and defender of quaternions, published the first edition of his *Elementary Treatise on Quaternions* in 1867. The first chapter of this book does not use the full quaternions, only the vector part, just as in a modern book on vector analysis. There was a second edition of the *Treatise* in 1873 and a third edition in 1890. In 1880 there was a German translation of Tait's book. The three editions of Tait's book are a good indication of the importance of his work in the history of vector analysis. He had a particular interest in the physical application of vector analysis.

Herman Grassmann published his *Ausdehnungslehre* (Theory of Extension) in 1844. This work, independently of Hamilton, developed the concepts of directed lines in space not only in two or three dimensions but for *n*-dimensions (Hamilton's quaternions were for space of three dimensions only). But Hamilton used the concept of steps in time, i.e. vectors in the one dimension of time. Hamilton also commented that Grassmann used the expression $B-A$ to represent the directed line or vector from A to B exactly in the same way as Hamilton himself had done. Oliver Heavyside also made important contributions to vector analysis, developing his system from those of Hamilton and Tait by elimination and simplification. Heavyside used vector analysis for physical applications, especially to electricity. He published a lengthy exposition of his vectorial system in his *Electromagnetic Theory* in 1893, in which he tells the story of a boy who studied Hamilton's quaternions but found the property wholly incomprehensible. How could the square of a vector be negative?

Heavyside has a very important comment on quaternions:

> The quaternions and its laws were discovered by that extraordinary genius Sir W. Hamilton. A quaternion is neither a scalar nor a vector, but a sort of combination of both. It has no physical representatives, but is a highly abstract mathematical concept.[7]

Hamilton's quaternions are an extension of the concept of vectors from the two dimensions of a plane to the three dimensions of space. It would therefore be very surprising if it had no physical representation or application. After considerable study and thought I have developed the theory that the vectors i, j, k are the axes of a body subject to spin, i.e. intrinsic angular momentum. Bodies subject to spin include tops, gyroscopes, the earth and the other planets, and atomic particles, e.g. electrons. The axes of bodies subject to spin are indeed imaginary in experience as well as algebraically: thus i, j, k are all imaginary, their squares are equal to -1. But the vectors in vector analysis are real, their squares are positive. This problem has been discussed by one of the most important defenders of Hamilton's quaternions, Cargill Gilston Knott, during the debates between the supporters of quaternions and the vector analysts. Knott read an important paper, 'Recent Innovations in Vector Theory', published in the proceedings of the Royal Society of Edinburgh in 1892:

Knott turned to the question of why the square of a unit vector should be equal to −1 . . . Thus a necessary condition for the associative law is that the square of a unit vector be equal to minus one. Knott made an issue of this, and it is not a small point.[8]

The next page of this source describes Knott's disagreement with the Heavyside–Gibbs–MacFarlane contention that the square of a vector should be positive. This disagreement was not only evident in Knott's use of the word 'assumption' to describe the work of these authors, but also ran through his whole paper. MacFarlane responded by arguing (correctly) that both views were assumptions (or, more correctly, definitions) and were completely arbitrary algebraically.[9]

In Thomas Hankins' biography of Hamilton the author states that by 1893 the battle between the quaternionists and the vector analysts was in full swing. It was really two battles: one of quaternions versus coordinates, and a second one of quaternions versus vectors. The first battle had begun as soon as quaternions appeared, but the second began only in 1890, after vector analysis became widely known. These differing views are related to the problem of the square of a vector being negative in quaternions and positive in vector analysis. In the one school of thought there are vectors with coordinates in vector analysis, and in the other vectors without coordinates, as with the quaternions. In each case the rotation of vectors is involved, but there are two different ways this rotation can be carried out. This can be shown by means of a simple diagram:

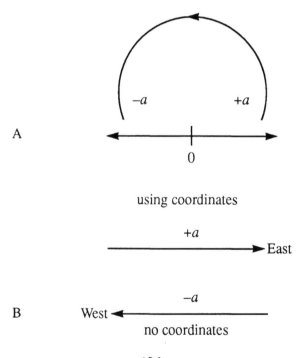

In diagram A the vector is rotated through 180°: this represents the motion of translation. In diagram B the vector +a represents the axis of spin, e.g. of a gyroscope, in the direction east and the vector −a is the reversal of the axis of spin to the direction west. The vector +a has left-handed spin, whereas the reversal of vector to −a reverses the direction of spin to right-handed.

In his biography of Hamilton Thomas Hankins gives an excellent account of the differences in mathematical operations between quaternions and the vectors of vector analysis. These differences clearly show the superiority from a purely mathematical point of view of quaternions over vector analysis:

> The multiplication of quaternions obeys all the rules of ordinary algebra except the commutative law. The multiplication of vectors on the other hand fails miserably on many counts. In the first place there are two kinds of multiplication in vector analysis, a condition that would have distressed Hamilton. The dot product of two vectors is not even a vector. Therefore the law of closure fails. The law of the moduli also fails, and therefore division is ambiguous. The cross product of two vectors is a vector and therefore the property of closure is maintained, but it does not satisfy either the commutative or the associative law and the law of the moduli fails as well. Also both products can be zero even when the factors are both finite, a condition that Hamilton especially wished to avoid. It is not surprising then that he did not develop vector analysis, although he certainly recognised many of its important properties. Vector analysis proved its worth in physics, and since Hamilton always postponed investigating the applications of quaternions while he worked on the algebra he was unlikely to develop vector analysis as a practical method.[10]

Cornelius Lanczos gives an excellent account of the differences between Herman Grassmann's algebra which its author called *Ausdehnungslehre* – i.e. the Theory of Extension – published in 1844 and Hamilton's quaternions, clearly showing the mathematical superiority of the quaternions.

> Grassmann's ideas were of too great generality but it was he who first introduced 'the inner product' – now called 'Scalar product' – of the two vectors, and 'Outer product' – now called 'Vector product' – of two vectors. Furthermore, the entire scheme of tensor calculus fits easily into Grassmann's calculus. We may wonder how that is possible in view of our previous claim that Hamilton's quaternions are the *only* example of a non-commutative algebra. The answer is that Grassmann's algebra is less complete than Hamilton's, because he sacrificed not only the commutative law of multiplication but another commonly accepted postulate of algebra according to which the zero has no factors. If the product of two numbers gives zero this is only possible if at least one of the two factors is zero. This is true also in Hamilton's algebra. It does not hold, however, in Grassmann's algebra, where the product of two numbers may come out as zero, although neither of the two numbers vanishes. Under such conditions the operation of division has to be sacrificed. In Grassmann's algebra we can add, subtract and multiply, but we cannot divide. In Hamilton's algebra all the four operations of algebra exist: addition, and subtraction, multiplication and division.[11]

127

The multiplication of quaternions is also associative. This was especially emphasised by Cargill Gilston Knott, who stated that a necessary condition for the associative law is that the square of a unit vector be equal to minus one. Hamilton has a special reference to and comments on Grassmann's *Ausdehnungslehre*. He noted the use of non-commutative multiplication. In ordinary algebra $ab = ba$, but there are algebras where $ab = -ba$, as in quaternions and Grassmann's work. Hamilton commentated that the symbol $B-A$ used by Grassmann to denote a directed line from A to B is exactly the same as his own use of the same symbolism. The directed line is called *Strecke* in German – which means a stretch, and which Hamilton called a vector, from the Latin *vehere*, to carry, i.e. the point from A to B. The word *Strecke* meaning stretch is a useful alternative to vector. It could be applied to a stretch of road or the stretch of a river between two points. It is at once evident that you can have the stretch in the opposite direction, and that the progression in each direction could be different, i.e. not equal. The stretch on the road could be uphill or against the wind, in which case the stretch in opposite direction would be different. The stretch on the river could be with the flow of the river or against the flow, with an obvious and important difference. In the same reference Hamilton says that Grassmann was not in possession of the theory of quaternions, and that in the preface to the book he (Grassmann) stated that he had not succeeded in extending the use of imaginaries from the plane to space and did not succeed in constructing a theory of angles in space.[12]

Although there is a comprehensive account of vector analysis including Hamilton's quaternions in Michael Crowe's *History of Vector Analysis* there is no reference to some important mathematicians. Thirteen years after Hamilton's death G. Frobenius proved that there exist precisely three associative division algebras over the reals, namely the real numbers themselves, the complex numbers and the real quaternions – Frobenius' work on this was published in 1879.

Adolph Hurvitz (1859–1919) proved that algebras over the reals without zero divisors exist in dimensions 1, 2, 4 and 8. The reals of dimensions 1 and the complex numbers of dimension 2 are the only commutative and associative division algebras. The quaternions are a non-commutative associative division algebra of dimension 4. The Cayley algebra of dimension 8 is non-commutative and non-associative.

Michael Crowe in the preface to his book *A History of Vector Analysis* (1967) states that it is the first book on the subject. This is not entirely correct as an excellent book on vectors by Parry Moon and Domina Spencer was published in 1965.[13] The introduction to this book gives a brief account of the development of vector analysis referring to all the principal mathematicians involved, i.e. Hamilton, Grassmann, Gibbs and Heavyside. There is a set of four photographs of these mathematicians with the caption 'The Originators'. There are 38 references at the end of the historical introduction giving most of the important primary figures involved and some of the secondary sources, such as Felix Klein. At the end of the book, in Appendix A, there is a comprehensive list of 63 textbooks on vectors. One of the books listed is *Vector Analysis and Quaternions* by A. MacFarlane, published by John Wiley & Sons of New York in 1906. MacFarlane, together with Gibbs and Heavyside, insisted that the square of a vector should be positive, and not negative as in the quaternion calculus. (It is most fundamental that the square of the vectors should be negative in the quaternion.) About 1900 an International Association for Promoting the Study of Quaternions and Allied Systems of Mathematics was founded. A *Bulletin of the International Association* was published from 1900, the last issue appearing in 1913. MacFarlane was the general secretary of the Association and he became its real leader. In 1904 came the publication of a *Bibliography of Quaternions and Allied Systems of Mathematics*, which contained references to 2,500 articles in the vectorial tradition. It is very remarkable that MacFarlane, who was the leader and chief promoter of Hamilton's quaternions from 1900 to 1906, should have rejected one of the fundamental elements of the calculus, namely that the square of a vector should be positive, and not negative as in the formula $i^2 = j^2 = k^2 = -1$. In the vector analysis of Gibbs and Heavyside the square of vectors is positive: $i^2 = j^2 = k^2 = +1$. This is a good example of the difficulty of understanding the meaning of quaternions when we have the chief promoter and defender of quaternions explicitly rejecting a fundamental element of the calculus and making it the same as if the vector analysis formula was positive when it should be negative. We can then ask the question: what difference is there between the squares of i, j, k being positive and their being negative?

The vectors i, j, k represent in vector analysis the position of a body in space of three dimensions and, of course, of a body in motion in space. The vectors are coordinates using a frame of reference. The motion of the body in space is relative motion – relative to the frame of reference of the coordinates. In my special interpretation of quaternions, the vectors i, j, k, whose squares are -1 – i.e. they are imaginary – represent the one axis of a body subject to spin or intrinsic angular momentum. These vectors are not coordinates – they do not give the position of the body in space, no frame of reference is required. The body is in the same place all the time, e.g. a spinning top or gyroscope. The vectors i, j, k of quaternions represent the axis of spin in the three directions of the space of the real natural world, i.e. north–south, east–west and up and down:

$+i$ – East	$+j$ – North	$+k$ – Up
$-i$ – West	$-i$ – South	$-k$ – Down

Spin has the unique property of having its motion in two and only two directions, i.e. right-handed and left-handed, or in other language clockwise or anticlockwise. When the direction of the axis is reversed from plus to minus the direction of the spin is reversed. Giving one example:

+k – axis upwards – left-handed spin
−k – axis downwards – right-handed spin

The word 'rotation' is ambiguous, as it can be used for either spin or orbital angular momentum, e.g. the earth is both rotating on its axis *and* rotating in orbit around the sun – it has the two motions. The motion of spin is not relative to any frame of reference, for the motion is absolute – no coordinates are required. The vectors i, j, k of the quaternions represent the directions of the axis of spin – there is no motion of the body from place to place, since a body subject to spin remains in the same place. As already shown the rotation of vectors can be done in two different ways:

1   For the position of a body in space and its motion of translation from place to place:

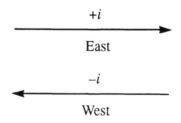

0

2   For the reversal of the axis of spin:

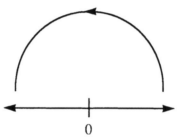

In the case of spin the vector is reversed in its own length – it is rotated around its midpoint and there is no change of position of the body subject to the motion of spin. It is worth repeating what Heavyside has said about a quaternion, namely that it is neither a scalar nor a vector but a sort of combination of both, and has no physical representatives. (It is in fact hard to believe that it has no physical representation after such elaborate study and development for so many years by Hamilton.) My interpretation that *i, j, k* represent the axis of spin still leaves open the interpretation of the full quaternion, which is quadruple algebra:

$$q = a + ib + jc + kd$$

In this formula, *a* is the scalar part and *ib + jc + kd* is the vector part. As already described, the scalar part can usefully be given as *s*. Hamilton, after some doubt and hesitation, thought the scalar part of the quaternion should represent time. He expressed this point of view in a poem, 'The Tetractys', written for Herschel in 1846:

and how the One Of Time, Of Space The Three,
might in the chain of Symbol, girdled be.[14]

This is a theory of time–space. In the set four numbers of the quaternion time is the first number, the scalar part, while the remaining three numbers are the vector part of the quaternion. The triple algebra of vector analysis is obviously obtained by removing or cancelling the first symbol, the scalar, so that there is no symbol for time remaining. The triplets or triple algebra which Hamilton had such difficulty in multiplying are obtained by removing the fourth symbol – *kd* – from the quaternion *a + ib + jc + kd*.

If *d* is 0 you have *a + ib + jc*, which was the triplet which Hamilton thought sufficient for rotations in space of three dimensions. If *c* is 0 you are left with *a + ib*, the complex number – a vector in two-dimensional space. If *b, c* and *d* are each 0, the scalar or real number remains. This simple method shows the mathematical elegance and comprehensiveness of quaternions. It would be amazing if they had no practical use or value, but only historical interest. Vector analysis is a triple algebra derived from the quadruple algebra of quaternions. The question remains: what is the meaning of the full set of four numbers that make up the quadruple algebra of quaternions? I have given the answer with my interpretation of quaternions: the symbols *i, j, k* represent the three axes of a body subject to spin – they are vectors whose squares equal –1, i.e. they are all imaginary. They represent the imaginary axes of a body subject to spin, e.g. a gyroscope. The very concept of spin, which is a very special type of motion, requires time. The symbol for time is the first one of the quaternion – the scalar part, represented by *a* at the beginning of the alphabet or *w* at the end of the alphabet, or more properly using *s* (for 'scalar'). The scalar number for time – the first symbol of the quaternion – is according to Hamilton extra-spatial or non-spatial and can be represented by a horizontal line extending in theory between + infinity and – infinity:

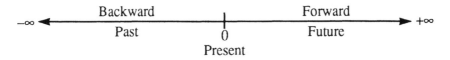

Time has two directions only: forward to the future and backward to the past. Hamilton took it for granted that the scalar number extended to infinity in each direction. The motion of spin has the unique property of having only two directions, right-handed and left-handed. There appears to be a correlation here with time, which also has two and only two directions. The vectors i, j, k represent the three directions of Euclidean space – north–south, east–west and up–down.

I will now set out the differences between quaternions and vector analysis in two columns:

Quaternions	Vector analysis
Quadruple algebra	Triple algebra
$a + ib + jc + kd$	i, j, k
a = scalar part or time part	No time part, only vector part
$ib + jc + kd$ = vector part	
Coordinate-free	With coordinates
Restricted to three dimensions	Can be extended to spaced n-dimension (Grassmann)
i, j, k are all imaginary	i, j, k are all real
$i^2 = j^2 = k^2 = -1$	$i^2 = j^2 = k^2 = +1$

Operations of algebra

Quaternions	Vector analysis
1 Associative for addition and multiplication	Associative not possible
2 Division possible	Division not possible
3 Multiplication non-commutative	Vector product or cross-product are non-commutative
Multiplication has one operation	Multiplication has two operations: a) scalar or dot product b) vector or cross-product
4 Law of the moduli	Law of the moduli fails

Significant interpretations

Quaternions	Vector analysis
1st symbol of the quadruple algebra a, w or s represents time – i.e. scalar part	No symbol for time in triple algebra
Vector part i, j, k represents the axes of a body subject to spin in three dimensions of space	Vectors i, j, k represent position and motion of a body in space of three dimensions
In e.g. tops, gyroscope or spin of earth and other planets motion of spin is absolute	In motion of body in space motion of translation is relative
No frame of reference required, no coordinates required	Frame of reference using coordinates required

The most important interpretation of quaternions is the representation of i, j, k as the axes of a body subject to spin. This is not merely the rotation of the axis of a rigid body, but of a body which must be spinning, which is a motion in time. It is important to enquire if Hamilton considered the application of quaternions to the problem of rotation or spin. There are some references to this in Volume 3 of his *Mathematical Papers*:

> Some valuable papers on couples, Quaternions and Octaves, have also been communicated to the same magazine [*Philosophical Magazine*] since the commencement of 1845 by Arthur Cayley Esq. especially on application of quaternions (which appeared in the February of that year) to the representation of the rotation of a solid body. That important application of the author's principles had indeed occurred to himself previously; but he was happy to see it handled by one so well versed as Mr Cayley is in the theory of such rotation and possessing such entire command of the resources of algebra and of geometry.[15]

The problem of rotation is again mentioned by Hamilton in one of his most important articles, communicated to the Royal Irish Academy in November 1844. In this paper, 'Quaternions: Geometrical Illustrations', he discussed the fourth proportional to three rectangular lines when the directions of those lines are taken into account. This line representing the fourth proportional is extra-spatial and has two directions, forward and backward. The line is also on a scale from negative to positive infinity, which led Hamilton to consider that it represents time which is not three-dimensional but unidimensional. This is of course the scalar part, the first part of the quaternion. Hamilton then goes on to consider rotations:

> Again, let us consider the more difficult problem of the composition of any number of successive rotations of a body, or at first, of any one line thereof, round several successive axes, through any angles small or large.[16]

A footnote again refers to Arthur Cayley's discovery of a formula which represents rotations.

In Chapter 3, Section 21 of the *Mathematical Papers* there is a special paper communicated in January 1848, entitled 'On Quaternions and the Rotation of a Solid Body'.[17] At the end of Volume 3 of this collection of Hamilton's papers is Appendix I, compiled by the editors, on 'Quaternions and Rotations'[18], with several references to work done in this field by A.W. Conway and Cornelius Lanczos and several others. There is again a reference to Cayley's paper 'On Certain Results Relating to Quaternions', with the formula for a rotation.

Hamilton's quaternions are used in the classic treatise *Über die Theorie des Kreisels* (On the Theory of Tops) by Klein and Somerfeld to give simple and elegant means of representing rotations in space. This also applies to the theory of the gyroscope. E.T. Whittaker has pointed out that the spin-matrices introduced by Pauli in 1927 on which the quantum mechanical theory of rotations and angular momenta depends are simply Hamilton's three quaternion units i, j, k.

I would now like to give a list of mathematicians whose work in books or articles I have used in my efforts to understand the meaning and application of Hamilton's quaternions and vector analysis:

1 William Rowan Hamilton
2 Robert Percival Graves
3 Thomas Hankins
4 Sean O'Donnell
5 Peter Guthrie Tait
6 Herman Grassmann
7 Arthur Cayley
8 C.G. Knott
9 A. MacFarlane
10 G. Frobenius
11 Adolf Hurwitz
12 Felix Klein
13 Josiah Willard Gibbs
14 Oliver Heavyside
15 E.T. Bell
16 Michael Crowe
17 Reginald Stephenson
18 Arthur W. Conway
19 Cornelius Lanczos
20 B.L. Van der Waerden
21 Rev. P.J. McLaughlin
22 George Temple
23 E.T. Whittaker
24 Don M. Yost
25 Alfred Bork
26 G.J. Whitrow
27 L.E. Dickson
28 J.L. Synge
29 J.C. Maxwell
30 C.C. MacDuffee.

On the last page of the chapter on Hamilton and quaternions in Michael Crowe's *A History of Vector Analysis*, the author gives his final opinion: 'There is something tragic in the thought of the brilliant Hamilton devoting the last twenty-two years of his life to quaternions which are now of little interest.' Earlier in the book the author had shown that quaternions in fact led to the development of vector analysis by Gibbs and Heavyside, so it is completely unacceptable for him to say that quaternions in themselves are of little interest. In the introduction to Volume 3 of Hamilton's *Mathematical Papers* the editors H. Halberston and R.E. Ingram give their final opinion that Hamilton's quaternions are a formidable mathematical edifice, the achievement of a mind of power, understanding and originality. Quaternions have a paramount significance both in mathematics and as a means of describing nature. In modern times several authors have proposed versions of quantum mechanics in which quaternions play a central part. Reference is given to Appendix I of Volume 3 of the *Mathematical Papers* on 'Quaternions and Rotations', which has already been mentioned.

We must now consider the application and use of quaternions in the philosophy of physics, or more correctly the philosophy of mathematical physics.

8 The unification of physics

The problem of the unification of physics is the most fundamental and final problem in physics. It is better to use the language and concept of 'unification' rather than the 'theory of everything', which suggests unifying all branches of knowledge including biology and human studies. We are only concerned with the unification of physics, or more exactly mathematical physics.

This problem can best be studied by beginning with an examination of the laws of nature. I have worked out a scheme to examine the whole subject in eight sections. They are listed very briefly as follows:

1 The laws of nature
2 The arrow of time
3 Einstein's special theory of relativity
4 Einstein's general theory of relativity, theory of gravitation
5 Quantum theory
6 Cosmology – the Big Bang and expansion of the universe
7 The philosophy of science – especially the philosophy of mathematics and its applications to nature
8 The relation between science and religion – the existence of a God or no God.

This is a very comprehensive list: a book could be written on each of the eight sections. But by considering the most fundamental aspects of each section, the account can be quite brief. The problem of unification will be limited to the two most fundamental branches of physics – gravitation theory and quantum theory. Einstein's special theory of relativity was published in

1905 and the general theory in 1915. The dates of the quantum theory are Planck in 1900, Bohr in 1913, Heisenberg in 1925, and Schrödinger in 1926.

It is clear that the full quantum theory was not developed until 1925/26. The discovery of the spin of the electron and other particles is especially important. These discoveries took place after Einstein's general theory of relativity in 1915 and are more fundamental. Therefore the central problem of the unification of physics is the application of quantum theory to gravitation theory. In spite of every effort to achieve this, it has so far not been successfully accomplished.

We begin with the laws of nature.

1 The laws of nature

Only the most fundamental and generalised laws are given. The following is the list of five laws as given in my book *The Logical Universe: The Real Universe* published in 1994, with slight modification:

1   The conservation laws
2   Symmetry
3   The laws of motion expressed as equations
4   The constancy of the speed of light
5   The uniformity of nature

The conservation laws include:

The conservation of mass
The conservation of mass/energy using Einstein's equation $E = MC^2$
The conservation of linear momentum
The conservation of angular momentum or spin.[1]

On examining these five laws it is evident that they are not five different laws, but in fact are all saying the same thing – that there is an invariance with respect to time. There is no change with the passage of time. Since there is no change with time, the laws do not give the initial conditions in the universe. In consequence of this invariance with time, there is no law which can give an age of the universe. The laws break down at any beginning of the universe.

John Barrow in his book *The World within the World* gives a beautiful account of the relation between symmetries and invariances and conservation:

The simplest and most important pairings of symmetries and invariances are given as follows:

137

The laws of nature invariant under the operation of:	Conserved quantity
Translations in space	Linear momentum
Translations in time	Energy
Rotations in space	Angular momentum

These beautiful relationships reveal the extent to which deep symmetry was unknowingly built into the laws of motion found by Newton. The principal conservation laws are consequences of the fact that the laws of nature do not depend upon the position, orientation or time at which they are observed.[2]

The word 'rotation' is ambiguous, as it could mean rotation as translation – e.g. the rotation of the earth around the sun – or rotation of a body on its axis – e.g. spin, which is also a motion of the earth, as well as of tops and gyroscopes. The angular momentum therefore has two forms: orbital angular momentum and intrinsic angular momentum or spin. In each case the invariance is a consequence of no essential change taking place with the progression or flow of time.

When you examine more closely the five laws of nature already given they are all valid for gravitation theory, but one law is not valid for quantum theory. The five laws are listed again for quantum theory:

1   The conservation laws.
2   Symmetry.
3   The equations of motion are not equal. They do not commute.
4   The constancy of the speed of light.
5   The uniformity of nature.

The laws are the same except for number 3. In gravitation theory the equations commute, but in quantum theory the equations do not commute, they are anticommuting. The algebra required is non-commutative. When the equations are equal the process of motion is continuous. When the equations do not commute it means the process of change has an element of discontinuity, an imprecision which is built into the theory. This radical difference of the two theories is a special problem for their unification. Gravitation theory is a continuous change but in quantum theory the change is discontinuous. These two states of affairs are contradictory, their unification is impossible. Einstein never accepted the discontinuous or statistical character of quantum theory; to express this point of view he used the expression 'God does not play dice', meaning that there is no element of chance or indeterminism in nature. It is obvious that unification of the two theories is impossible without some radical change.

The next problem to be considered is to ask why the laws of nature are as they are. This question has been asked by many scientists and philosophers of science, but it has been done most clearly and explicitly by Paul Davies in his book *God and the New Physics*. In the preface to the book the author states 'The central theme of the book concerns what I call the Big Four questions of existence: Why are the laws of nature what they are?'[3]

I give only the first of Davies' four questions – why are the laws of nature what they are? Unfortunately the author has no satisfactory answer to the question.

I believe the answer to this most important and fundamental question is given in the best book published on the philosophy of time, *The Natural Philosophy of Time* by G.J. Whitrow:

> Mathematically the origin – if any – of time is projected to 'minus infinity', which means that in practice it is irrelevant and only time differences matter. This irrelevance of the origin of time is directly associated with the fact that the time variable does not appear explicitly in the mathematical formulation of the fundamental laws of physics. Indirectly it is also associated with the fact that the laws of classical mechanics are reversible and do not distinguish between past and future. In classical mechanics there is no special epoch which can serve as a fundamental point of reference, with respect to which earlier and later can be distinguished. The second law of thermodynamics suggests the possibility of a terminal limiting points in the future, but as we have seen the cosmological application of this law is a disputed hypothesis. The difficulty does not absolve us however from the duty of considering the problem of a natural origin of time.[4]

This is really the same point of view as shown in the five laws of nature. They are in essence all the same, they express the invariance of the laws with respect to time. There is no fundamental change in physical nature with the passage or progression of time. The Big Bang theory of cosmology, which presupposes an expansion of the universe, provides an age for the universe. But there is no law of nature which can give an age for the universe, which seems very strange. Whitrow has given the explanation for this in the extract above. It is assumed that time extends to infinity in the past. But if time and the universe had a beginning in the past, some law of nature ought to provide that age. Everything depends on the nature and meaning of time, which will be considered in the next section.

2 The arrow of time

In any discussion of the nature and meaning of time, the clearest and simplest introduction to its study is to draw a diagram. This must be a horizontal line extending to right and left. As soon as this is done it is obvious that there are two possibilities: the line of time can be made to extend to infinity in the past or to a beginning of time.

In each case time has two directions, forward and backward. The moments

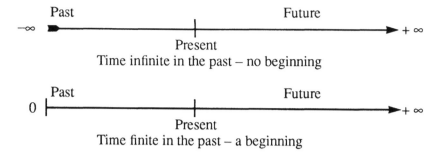

Time infinite in the past – no beginning

Time finite in the past – a beginning

or epochs of time are dates which are represented by numbers, e.g. 1925 or 1965. They are scalar numbers giving the measurement of time, i.e. they are the scalars of the real numbers. Hamilton first used the word 'scalar' to describe the scale of numbers from minus infinity to plus infinity. He described time as unidimensional and extra-spatial. He also used the term intensive magnitude rather than extensive magnitude. The word 'extensive' suggests extension – a spatial concept which Hamilton wished to avoid. The presence or absence of an arrow of time can be well summarised in six categories – four covering when it is present and two when it is absent, as shown in the following list:

Arrow of time

Present

1 Human experience
2 Biology
3 Thermodynamics
4 Expansion of the universe – cosmological arrow.

Absent

5 Classical mechanics
  Special theory of relativity
  General theory of relativity – gravitation theory
6 Quantum theory.

It is clearly evident that there is a flow of time in human experience – the future is not yet known, while the past is gone and only experienced as a memory. The whole of human life is based on the flow of time in one direction, the forward direction. For example, a war is planned, declared and fought, and soldiers are killed and buried. At the end peace is made and signed. If the flow of time is reversed the peace treaty is signed first, the soldiers rise from the dead, the bullets that killed them go back into their enemies' guns. Then all the soldiers go home and war is declared. All this could not happen in reality – the flow of time is in one direction and is irreversible. It is perhaps in biology that the arrow of time is most evident, with the birth of living beings, their growth, ageing and death, and of course the whole of evolution is a progression in one direction – its opposite would be nonsense. It is rather strange that Stephen Hawking in his book *A Brief History of Time* describes three arrows of time:

> There are at least three different arrows of time. First there is the thermodynamic arrow of time, the direction of time in which disorder of entropy increases. Then there is the psychological arrow of time. This is the direction in which we feel time passes, the direction in which we remember the past but not the future. Finally, there is the cosmological arrow of time. This is the direction of time in which the Universe is expanding rather than contracting.[5]

It is surprising that Hawking does not mention the arrow of time in biology when it is so clear and evident and the consequences of the reversal of time are so obviously impossible in reality.

In the first section on the laws of nature it was established that the concepts of conservation and symmetry were dependent on the assumption of the infinity of time in the past. Time is symmetric if it had no beginning. If time had a beginning it would be asymmetric, i.e. it would have an arrow. Time with no beginning has no arrow. These are two radically different states which can be usefully represented in a double column:

Table of time	
Time with no beginning	Time with a beginning
No arrow	An arrow
Symmetric	Asymmetric
Directionless, or in	With direction, or in
German *Zeitrichtunglos*	German *Zeitrichtung*
Isotropic	Anisotropic

There are four different concepts of time each of which has its opposite state of affairs. Thus for the arrow there is either a flow of time in one direction or no flow of time. Symmetric time means there is no difference between past and future, whereas with asymmetric time there is a difference between past and future. The word 'direction' suggests a forward flow of time and 'directionless' that there is no flow of time. The last concept given is the most accurate and comprehensive, and extends the notion of direction. The word 'isotropic' means the same in each direction, of which there are two and only two, forward and backward. That is, forward and backward in time are the same, there is no flow and no arrow. The negative form of this word, 'anisotropic', means time is not the same in each direction; again there are only two directions, forward and backward, to the future and to the past. This is perfectly obvious in human life and in biology – even the youngest child could understand the difference. We must now consider the concept of dimensions and directions in time and compare it with the same concept in space.

Time has one dimension, best represented by a horizontal line extending forward and backward. The times or dates are scalars – the real number system. Euclidean space has three dimensions – the depth, the length and the height. Time has two directions – forward and backward, to the future and to the past. Space has three basic directions – north–south, east–west, and up–down. There are innumerable intermediate directions in space – e.g. north-west, north-east, etc. All the directions in space are the same, they are isotropic. Hamilton frequently refers to the fact that the different directions in space are equivalent. His formula for quaternions

$$i^2 = j^2 = k^2 = -1$$

expresses the isotropic character of Euclidean space. The direction for i (east–west), j (north–south) and k (up and down) are all equal. A simple diagram will show these distinctions very clearly:

TIME	SPACE
1 dimension	3 dimensions
2 directions	3 directions

There are two categories of motion in natural phenomena. In the motion of translation, bodies move from place to place and have three basic directions. With the motion of spin, the body – e.g. a top or gyroscope – is not moving from place to place, there is no translation. The body is in motion, spinning on an axis which is pointing in one direction. The motion has two and only two directions, left-handed and right-handed. As has already been affirmed on several occasions, time has two and only two directions, exactly the same as the motion of spin. There thus appears to be a correlation between time and the motion of spin as each has only two directions. This is not the case with the motion of translation as this has basically three directions and time has only two – here the correlation is absent.

3 Einstein's special theory of relativity

Einstein published his special theory of relativity in June 1905. The fundamental assumption of the whole theory is that motion is of bodies from place to place – a motion of translation. The purpose of mechanics is to describe how bodies change their position in space with time. A good example of motion is that of trains and railway carriages which are travelling uniformly. We call such motions a uniform translation (uniform because it is of a constant velocity and direction) translation because although the carriage changes its position relative to the track yet it does not rotate in so doing). To describe a motion of translation a frame of reference is required, expressed by coordinates which are vectors.

The speed of light is independent of the motion of the observer – i.e. the motion of translation. This is implied by Maxwell's equations in which the speed of light is constant. Bodies contract with increasing speed and clocks run slow. The magnitude of these changes can be calculated by the formulae of Lorentz transformations. The special theory of relativity can be concisely expressed in two postulates:

1   The laws of physics take the same form in all inertial frames.
2   In any given inertial frame, the speed of light is the same whether the light is emitted by a body at rest or by a body in uniform motion of translation.

The space of special relativity is Euclidean and there is no gravitational field present. This appears to be an unreal and unnatural state of affairs. In reality the influence of gravity is always present.

Owing to the finite speed of light it is impossible to ascertain the simultaneity of events. As a direct consequence of the special theory of relativity the concept of absolute universal time is abolished. Each frame of reference has its own time. There are as many times as there are inertial frames. The concept of absolute space is also abolished: each observer has his own space and frame of reference. This radical change can be called a revolution. There is the change from the absolute space and time of Newton to a relative space and time. Ian Stewart in his recent book *From Here to Infinity* has a curious observation about the theory of relativity:

> When Einstein's Theory of Relativity achieved public recognition most people interpreted it as saying that 'everything is relative', a comfortable philosophy that, for example, justifies the ignoring the poor on the ground that others are poorer. However, that's not what Einstein was saying; he was telling us that the speed of light is not relative, but absolute. It should have been named the theory of non-Relativity.[6]

This interpretation of Einstein's special relativity is not acceptable. It is perfectly correct to speak of the non-relativity of the speed of light – this speed is assumed to be constant and absolute – but the 'relativity' of the theory refers to the motion of the translation, which is the type of motion described. This is relative to a frame of reference and is expressed by coordinates x, y, z for three-dimensional Euclidean space. The 'theory of relativity' is the perfectly correct terminology to use.

Herman Minkowski made a most important contribution to the mathematical formulation of the special theory of relativity:

> There [University of Göttingen] on November 5 1907, he gave a colloquium about relativity in which he identified Lorentz transformations with pseudo-rotations for which $X_1^2 + X_2^2 + X_3^2 + X_4^2$ is invariant, $X_4 = ict$ where X_1, X_2, X_3 denote the spatial variables.[7]

The X_4 variable is for time. Since it is expressed as ct it is a distance – a spatial variable – and since it is multiplied by $\sqrt{-1}$ or i it is rotated through 90° and is represented by a vertical line. This is the imaginary time coordinate, the fourth coordinate of Minkowski's four-dimensional space–time. The title of Chapter XVII of Einstein's book *Relativity: The Special and General Theory* is 'Minkowski's Four Dimensional Space'. There is no reference to time in that title. Time has been spatialised: it is represented by an imaginary time coordinate ict – the fourth dimension. In diagrams this is represented by a vertical line which emphasises the spatial character of the time coordinate. Minkowski published a detailed paper soon after the colloquium at Göttingen. Terms such as 'spacelike vector', 'timelike vector', 'light cone' and 'world line' stem from this paper.

At first Einstein was not impressed with Minkowski's mathematical formulation of the special theory. He called it *Überflussige Gelehrsamkeit* (superfluous learnedness). However, he later accepted Minkowski's contribution to his theory, especially as it greatly facilitated the transition from special to general relativity. Minkowski's famous address on 'Space and Time' was given at Cologne on 21 September 1908. The first short paragraph is quoted from Pais' book on Einstein:

> The views of space and time which I wish to lay before you have sprung from the soil of experimental physics, and therein lies its strength. They are radical. Henceforth space by itself, and time by itself, are doomed to fade away into mere shadows, and only a kind of union of the two will preserve an independent reality.[8]

The union of space and time is achieved by making time the fourth dimension of space – although imaginary, it is the fourth coordinate. Minkowski's space–time is a four-dimensional model of physical space and time: formally a space in which three coordinates specify the position of a point in space and the fourth coordinate represents the time at which an event occurs at that point. The three coordinates giving the position of a point or body in space are vectors and can be used to describe the change of position in space, i.e. a motion of transition relative to a frame of reference. The fourth coordinate X_4 – i.e. ict – is imaginary and represents time by a line which is vertical. This is shown in a simple diagram:

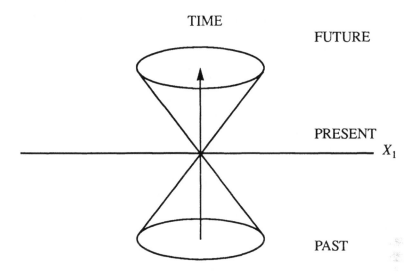

TIME

FUTURE

PRESENT X_1

PAST

In any normal diagram of time a line is drawn horizontally:

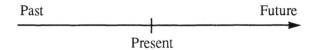

Past   Future

Present

This clearly indicates the two directions of time: forward to the future and backward to the past. Looking at the horizontal line, the future is to the right and the past to the left of the point which represents the present. To make a time diagram with the line upwards and downwards is to represent time spatially, which is what the theory of relativity has done. The three coordinates for space X_1, X_2, X_3 are vectors which are real – their squares are positive. The fourth coordinate representing time is also a vector, but it is imaginary – the square of the vector is negative $(ict)^2 = -c^2t^2$. Minkowski's space–time is represented by a set of four numbers, i.e. quadruple algebra. Three are vectors for space and one the vector for time, i.e. the numbers represent four vectors – this is mentioned by Einstein when he refers to 'an arbitrary inertial system of the X_1, X_2, X_3, X_4 is called a 4-vector'.[9]

The mathematical formulation of Minkowski's space–time can be summarised in a simple diagram:

MINKOWSKI'S SPACE–TIME Quadruple algebra – 4 vectors	
SPACE	TIME
3 vectors	1 vector
All real	Imaginary
Their square is positive	The square is negative

One of the most important consequences of Einstein's special theory of relativity is that involving the concept of time. A revolution has taken place: absolute time is abolished, time is now relative to each observer's frame of reference. The concept of a flow of time and an arrow of time is totally absent.

G.J. Whitrow's *The Natural Philosophy of Time* is probably the most valuable and comprehensive book on the whole subject. The beginning of its first chapter is called 'Elimination of Time' – meaning the absence of a flow of time and of a direction of time in physics. The following quotation is an excellent summary of Whitrow's critique:

> In mathematical physics, Lavoisier's contemporary Lagrange was the forerunner of Minkowski and Einstein in affirming that time could be regarded as a fourth dimension of space. He realised that the time variable of a rational mechanics based on Newton's laws of motion does not point in a unique direction and that in principle, all motions and dynamical processes subject to these laws are reversible, just like the ones of a geometrical co-ordinate system. Moreover, the origin of Newtonian time can be as freely and arbitrarily chosen as can the origin of a Cartesian co-ordinate system. By regarding physical time as a fourth dimension of space, Lagrange all but eliminated time from dynamical theory. The 'Elimination' of time from natural philosophy is closely correlated with the influence of geometry . . . Galileo's great achievements in dynamics were largely due to his successful exploitation of the device for representing time by a geometrical straight line. The primary object of Einstein's profound researches on the forces of nature has been well epitomised in the slogan 'the geometrization of physics', time being completely absorbed into the geometry of a hyperspace. Thus, instead of ignoring the temporal aspect of nature as Archimedes did, post-Renaissance mathematicians and physicists have to explain it away in terms of the spatial, and in this they have been aided by philosophers, notably the idealists.[10]

As well as the absolute character of time being eliminated in special relativity, any idea of the flow of time in one direction has also been eliminated. The motion of translation is relative. I see no objection to representing time by a geometrical straight line providing the line is horizontal, so that it can represent time forward to the right – the future – and backward to the left – the past. This is more suggestive of the extra-spatial character of time. If the line representing time is vertical it is given a spatial character, as in the Minkowski diagram shown earlier.

We will now consider the critical comments of a more recent study on time, namely Paul Davies' book *About Time* with its subtitle 'Einstein's Unfinished Revolution'. In the prologue the author comments:

> For a start, Einstein's time has no arrow; it is blind to the distinction between past and future. Certainly it does not *flow* like the time of Shakespeare or James Joyce, or for that matter of Newton. It is easy to conclude that something vital remains missing. Some extra quality to time left out of the equations, or that there is more

than one *sort* of time. The revolution begun by Einstein remains frustratingly unfinished.[11]

and again:

> Attempts to explain the flow of time using physics, rather than trying to define it away using philosophy, are probably the most exciting contemporary developments in the study of time. Elucidating the mysterious flux would, more than anything else, help unravel the deepest of all scientific enigmas – the nature of the human self. Until we have a firm understanding of the flow of time or incontrovertible evidence that it is indeed an illusion, then we will not know who we are, or what part we are playing in the great cosmic drama.[12]

And finally Davies expresses the problem in a very neat phrase: 'In my opinion, the greatest outstanding riddle concerns the glaring mismatch between physical time and subjective or psychological time.'[13]

The word 'mismatch' explains the problem perfectly. There is a radical difference between the time of physics – both in gravitation theory and quantum theory – and time as a human subjective experience. But the flow of time and the arrow of time are an objective phenomenon in living beings. Living beings grow and age and die at the end of life. At the beginning life commences with birth. To consider the progression of all these phenomena in the reverse order is totally unreal: the same flow of time in one direction is fundamental to the evolution of living beings. It seems surprising that the biologists are not complaining of the absence of this phenomenon in physics. They should be asking: why is there no arrow of time in physics?

To solve this most fundamental problem in physics I will develop a new theory.

A new theory of time–space and motion

John Barrow in his book *The World Within The World* gives a clear summary of the fundamental theses of Einstein's theory of relativity:

> ... Everyone, perhaps, except Albert Einstein, whose development of the special and general theories of relativity was to alter radically our picture of how the Universe works. The essential new ingredients from his theories and their experimental confirmation teach us a number of revolutionary lessons about the laws of nature:
>
> 1   Only relative motions are involved in the laws of nature.
> 2   There does not exist either an absolute space or an absolute time. They are different concepts for each observer in relative motion.[14]

I will only consider for the moment the first two summaries as given. The motion described by relativity is motion of translation, the motion of a body from place to place – a common example being the motion of trains. For motion of translation you require a frame of reference described by co-ordinates. But there is another type of motion which is well known in every-day experience and is most fundamental for physics. This is the motion of spin or intrinsic angular momentum. This is also called rotation but that term is ambiguous because it could also mean motion of translation in an orbit as well as motion around an axis, or spin. Spin bowling in cricket is standard practice – a twist is given to the ball to make it spin. In the game of snooker the ball is given spin very frequently by striking it off-centre with the cue. The standard example used to demonstrate the phenomenon of spin are tops and gyroscopes. As both tops and the simpler forms of gyroscope are toys, even children will be familiar with the phenomenon. The motion of spin is the most fundamental and universal in nature: the earth and all the planets and the moon are the subject of spin. In atomic theory the phenomenon of spin is universal: electrons and other elementary particles are subject to spin. There are two types of angular momentum: orbital – i.e. translation – and intrinsic – i.e. spin.

A body subject to spin is not moving from place to place – there is no translation, and no frame of reference is required for its description. The motion is not relative, it is absolute. It has the very special feature that spin is in two directions only, right-handed and left-handed. But the axis of spin has the three directions of Euclidean space, east–west, north–south, and up and down.

We will briefly consider the Copernican Revolution, which began with the publication of *De Revolutionibus Orbium Coelestium* in 1543, the year of Copernicus's death. In the Ptolemaic cosmology that prevailed before that date the earth was in the centre of the universe and had no motion. After the Copernican Revolution the earth had two motions – the translatory motion of its orbit around the sun, which was now the centre of the planetary system and the universe, and the rotation of the earth on its axis, or spin, explaining the daily rotation of the celestial sphere. For completeness there is a third motion – the wobble of the earth's axis, which is the cause of the precession of the equinoxes. After the Copernican Revolution, however, all study was concentrated on the motion of the earth in translation around the sun. When Galileo was alleged to have muttered 'None the less it does move' he was referring to the motion of translation only. When he observed the satellites of Jupiter they showed motion of translation. Newton, on the other hand, was convinced that there was absolute motion as well as relative motion, and to prove it used an experiment with a rotating bucket. When the bucket was rotated the water extended up the side of the bucket, and the water in the centre was at a lower level. By this experiment Newton was convinced that there was an absolute motion which could be demonstrated without the use of any frame of reference.

Foucault in Paris in 1851 demonstrated the rotation of the earth on its axis

– i.e. the spin of the earth – with his pendulum. In this device, a heavy weight is suspended by means of a fine wire from a considerable height, the plane of the swinging pendulum slowly changing with the rotation of the earth. This is the perfect demonstration of the spin of the earth on its axis and confirms Copernicus's theory. It seems remarkable that it took three hundred years – from 1543 to 1851 – to demonstrate this phenomenon. It seems that no one thought of doing it before then, not even the great Newton. This is a perfect demonstration of the absolute character of the motion of spin.

E.T. Whittaker, Professor of Mathematics at the University of Edinburgh and President of the Royal Society of Edinburgh, gave an important address on 'Spin in the Universe' at the Annual Statutory Meeting of the Society on 23 October 1944. Whittaker stated that rotation was a universal phenomenon, since the earth and all the other members of the solar system rotate on their axes. He described the discovery of spin in atomic theory:

> If we consider two frameworks of reference one of which is moving with a uniform velocity of translation relative to the other, then all the laws of nature have the same form with respect of the two frameworks. But the case is quite different with regard to rotations, a motion of rotation possessed by a system can be detected by observations taking place wholly within the system.[15]

For an example Whittaker mentions the rotating pail or bucket that Newton used. He then describes an optical experiment carried out in 1925 by Michelson and Gale by which they were able to deduce the angular velocity of the earth. He then concludes:

> Thus it is allowable to speak of velocities of rotation in an absolute manner, without the necessity of specifying any framework with respect to which the angular displacement takes place. The statement that some particular body is at rest as regards rotation is a statement that has meaning, although the statement that a particular body is at rest as regards translation is, taken by itself, meaningless.[15]

It is rather surprising that Whittaker does not mention Foucault's pendulum, which demonstrated the same absolute character of the spin of the earth as early as 1851. Foucault also used a specially mounted gyroscope to demonstrate the spin of the earth. We have now established without doubt the absolute character of the motion of spin, or intrinsic angular momentum.

Ernest Mach had considerable influence on Einstein, especially through his rejection of the concept of absolute motion:

> In his nineteenth century classic [*The Science of Mechanics*] Mach had indeed criticized the Newtonian view that one can distinguish between absolute and relative rotation. 'I cannot share this view. For me, only relative motions exist, and I can see, in this regard, no distinction between translation and rotation', he had written.[16]

The first paper written by Einstein (with Marcel Grossmann) on general relativity, published in 1913, contains several new touches concerning physics:

> First of all, Einstein takes a stand against Newton's argument for the absolute character of rotation (as demonstrated, for example by Newton's often reproduced discussion of the rotating bucket filled with water).[17]

In February 1916 Einstein gave a lecture on the Foucault pendulum. This is mentioned in Pais' biography but it is rather strange that there is no reference to Einstein's opinion of the experiment. I assume he did not accept that it was evidence for the absolute character of the motion of spin, and still believed that all motion was relative. We must now consider the number of dimensions of space. In Euclidean space, the space of the real natural world has three and only three dimensions – length, width and height, or east–west, north–south and up and down. John Barrow in his book *The World Within The World* has a valuable account of why physics requires only three dimensions:

1 Three dimensions are required for the stability of the orbital motion of the planets under the influence of gravitation.
2 Only in three dimensions can waves propagate in an undisturbed and reverberation-free fashion.
3 Perhaps most important of all: 'And only in three dimensions is the number of dimensions equal to the number of axes about which one can perform different rotations. This simple fact dictates the entire form of the laws of electromagnetism.'[18]

The phenomenon of spin takes place in three-dimensional Euclidean space. This space, like all space in the natural world, is subject to the influence of gravitation. This is especially evident in the phenomenon of precession, which occurs when a gyroscope is subjected to a force that tends to alter the direction of its axis: the gyroscope turns about an axis at right angles both to the axis about which the force was applied and to its main axis of spin.

Another property of the gyroscope is gyroscopic inertia – the direction of the axis of spin resists change so that it maintains the same orientation in space. This property forms the basis of the gyrocompass. This is a very different state of affairs compared to special relativity, for where there is an inertial non-accelerated frame of reference there is a total absence of gravity. As spin has three basic directions you require three numbers or symbols, one for each direction. Spin by its very nature is a motion which requires time, and hence another number or symbol – making four numbers, i.e. quadruple algebra.

We can now ask the question: what is the mathematics of spin, or intrinsic angular momentum? The answer must be Hamilton's quaternions. This answer should be evident to the reader after spending so much time and effort to understand the meaning and application of quaternions. The quadruple formula is:

$a + ib + jc + kd$ – using the first four letters of the alphabet
$w + ix + jy + kz$ – using the last four letters of the alphabet

Here, a and w are the scalar part. It is convenient to represent the scalar part by s:

$s + ia + jb + kc$

The vector part is $ia + jb + kc$:

$i_2 = j_2 = k_2 = -1$

Finally, i, j, k are the vectors which represent the three axes of spin:

$+i$ – east; $+j$ – north; $+k$ – up
$-i$ – west; $-j$ – south; $-k$ – down

Spin has only two directions, left and right – thus the spin direction of each symbol i, j, k is as follows:

$+i$ = left spin $+j$ = right spin $+k$ = left spin
$-i$ = right spin $-j$ = left spin $-k$ = right spin

The non-commutative multiplication of the vectors i, j, k is neatly given in three lines, A, B and C:

$i^2 = -1$	$j^2 = -1$	$k^2 = -1$	A
$ij = +k$	$jk = +i$	$ki = +j$	B
$ji = -k$	$kj = -i$	$ik = -j$	C

The order of multiplication reverses the direction of each axis and in consequence the direction of spin:

e.g. $ij = +k$ = left spin
      $ji = -k$ = right spin

Since i, j, k are the axes of spin, they are vectors whose squares are -1, therefore they are imaginary. The vectors are not coordinates, because they do not give the position of a body in space, they only give the direction of the axis in space. They could be called direction vectors.

In the quaternion $s + ia + jb + kc$, s – the scalar part – represents time, which can be shown in a diagram as a horizontal line. Time is represented by the first number in the quadruple formula. This is suggested by Hamilton's poem,

'And how the One of Time, Of Space the Three', written for Herschel in 1846. The poem was called 'The Tetractys', which is the Greek word for a set of four. The first symbol *s* in the quaternion formula is a scalar and represents time. For Hamilton the scalars are the real numbers of algebra:

> In short the *numbers* here spoken of, and elsewhere denominated '*scalars*' in this work, are simply those *positives* or *negatives* on the scale of progression from –∞ to +∞, which are commonly called *reals* (or real quantities) in algebra.[19]

The horizontal line representing time is a real number and is extra-spatial. This is very different from the Minkowski space–time formula, where time is the fourth dimension of space and the line representing it is vertical and imaginary. In quaternions the first number, the scalar representing time, can have two possibilities: it can extend to infinity in the past or have a beginning. If time had no beginning in the past it is symmetrical, and forward and backward are no different from one another. If time had a beginning, with 0 or zero at the beginning of the scale, then time is asymmetrical, i.e. it has an arrow, and forward and backward are different – it is not the same in each of the two directions. This is expressed in perfect and beautiful language – time is anisotropic. Symmetrical time – i.e. with no arrow – is the same in each direction – it is isotropic. We will assume that time had a beginning. The scale of time begins at 0 or zero – that makes it an absolute scale exactly analogous to the absolute scale of temperature, the Kelvin scale which begins at –273°C. By giving time a beginning we have introduced an arrow of time – i.e. asymmetric time or more correctly anisotropic time – into our theory of time–space. This essential character of time is totally absent in the special and general theories of relativity.

By making spin the fundamental motion we have returned to absolute motion, absolute – i.e. Euclidean – space and absolute time. This can be considered another Copernican Revolution. The first Copernican Revolution established the two basic motions of the earth, one of translation around the sun and the other the rotation or spin of the earth on its axis. Newton had accepted the absolute and universal flow of time. Einstein's theory of relativity made the motion of translation fundamental and abolished the absolute character of time. By basing the theory of time–space on the motion of spin which is absolute motion and making time a scalar with a beginning we have returned to absolute time. This is a second Copernican Revolution. This double revolution can be shown in three columns:

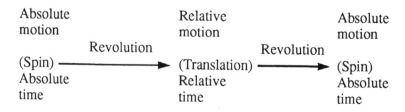

Absolute motion | Revolution | Relative motion | Revolution | Absolute motion
(Spin) ⟶ (Translation) ⟶ (Spin)
Absolute time | Relative time | Absolute time

Paul Davies in his recent book *About Time* (1995) refers to 'Einstein's Unfinished Revolution', and uses that expression as the subtitle of the book. Davies means that Einstein's theory of time is inadequate as it has no arrow, no directionality. However, the concept of an unfinished revolution is not satisfactory. A revolution is a change of one state of affairs to the contrary state of affairs. What is really required is another revolution – a return to the original state of affairs regarding motion and time as already described, using spin as the fundamental motion and Hamilton's quaternions as the quadruple algebra for representing time and space.

Roger Penrose has very relevant comments to make about the flow of time:

> In fact it is *only* the phenomenon of consciousness that requires us to think in terms of a 'flowing' time at all. According to relativity, one has just a 'static' four-dimensional space-time with no 'flowing' about it. The space-time is just *there* and time 'flows' no more than does space.[20]

Penrose has two very simple diagrams representing space and time:

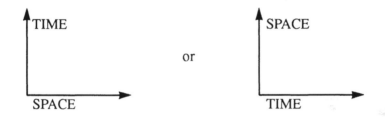

He says that there is nothing in the physicists' space–time that singles out time as something that flows. The first diagram with time vertical is Minkowski's space–time. Time is the fourth dimension of space and is imaginary. The whole theory is based on the motion of translation – the vertical line is a vector, the fourth vector.

The second diagram could represent the theory of time–space based on the motion of spin as already described. The horizontal line is a scalar, and if time has a beginning then the time is on an absolute scale. It is asymmetrical and has an arrow or, using the correct term, it is anisotropic – i.e. it is not the same in each direction, of which there are only two, forward and backward. The mathematical formulation of spin is Hamilton's quaternions. We will now summarise in a double column the differences between Minkowski's space–time and Hamilton's time–space based on his quaternion algebra.

As already mentioned, Einstein did not like Minkowski's mathematical formulation of the special theory of relativity. He called it 'superfluous learnedness'. But Hamilton's time–space as expressed in his quaternions based on the motion of spin could be considered greater learnedness or more learned and certainly not superfluous. The whole of Hamilton's representation of time–space is much superior to Einstein's special relativity. It has restored absolute time by basing the theory on the motion of spin and not that of translation. Gravitation is present whereas it is absent in special relativity, which is completely unreal. If time has a beginning it has an arrow, it is asymmetric and in the most correct terminology it is anisotropic – i.e. not the same in each of the two directions of time, forward and backward. This concept matches the time of human experience and biology.

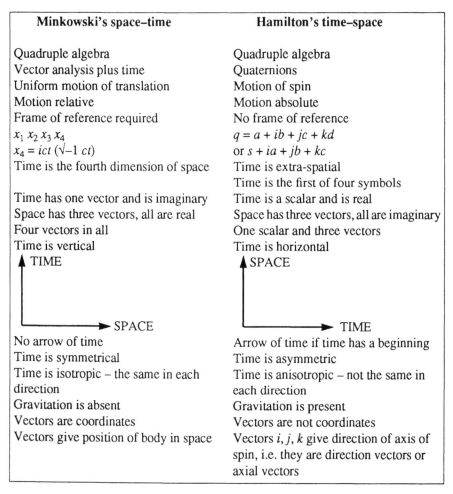

Minkowski's space–time	Hamilton's time–space
Quadruple algebra	Quadruple algebra
Vector analysis plus time	Quaternions
Uniform motion of translation	Motion of spin
Motion relative	Motion absolute
Frame of reference required	No frame of reference
$x_1\,x_2\,x_3\,x_4$	$q = a + ib + jc + kd$
$x_4 = ict\,(\sqrt{-1}\,ct)$	or $s + ia + jb + kc$
Time is the fourth dimension of space	Time is extra-spatial
	Time is the first of four symbols
Time has one vector and is imaginary	Time is a scalar and is real
Space has three vectors, all are real	Space has three vectors, all are imaginary
Four vectors in all	One scalar and three vectors
Time is vertical	Time is horizontal
(diagram: TIME vertical axis, SPACE horizontal axis)	(diagram: SPACE vertical axis, TIME horizontal axis)
No arrow of time	Arrow of time if time has a beginning
Time is symmetrical	Time is asymmetric
Time is isotropic – the same in each direction	Time is anisotropic – not the same in each direction
Gravitation is absent	Gravitation is present
Vectors are coordinates	Vectors are not coordinates
Vectors give position of body in space	Vectors i, j, k give direction of axis of spin, i.e. they are direction vectors or axial vectors

We must now consider the constancy of the speed of light, which is fundamental for the special theory of relativity. Ian Stewart in his recent book *From Here to Infinity* (1996) has very usefully pointed out that Einstein's theory could be called the theory of non-relativity because the speed of light is *not* relative but absolute. But of course the motion of translation is relative. There are two assumptions of the theory, one that the speed of light is absolute and motion is relative. The speed of light c is a universal constant – the value is 299,792,458 metres per second. This has been accepted as an exact measurement since 1983. In the special theory of relativity gravitation is absent – which is completely unrealistic. Since gravitation is a universal phenomenon and cannot be considered as non-existent, a change in the speed of light with time must be considered as an hypothesis. Is it certain that the speed of light will be exactly the same in 500 million years' time or was exactly the same 500 million years in the past? Dirac has considered changes in the constant of gravitation with time, so why not a change in the speed of light with time?

4 Einstein's general theory of relativity, theory of gravitation

Einstein's special theory of relativity of 1905 is only concerned with the uniform motion of translation in Euclidean space. The basic phenomenon of gravitation is acceleration. For Newton gravity was an attractive force acting at a distance, yet he gave no explanation of the cause and origin of this force which operated on the earth and was responsible for keeping all the planets in their orbits around the sun. Gravitation is therefore obviously a motion of translation. The gravitational field has a remarkable property: bodies which are moving under the influence of gravitation receive an acceleration which does not depend either on the material or on the physical state of the body. The gravitational mass of a body is equal to its inertial mass.

We are mainly concerned with Einstein's explanation of the phenomenon of gravitation. His full theory of general relativity with its mathematical formulation was not published until ten years after the special theory, in November 1915. It seems very remarkable that it took so long. The special theory is of uniform translatory motion in flat Euclidean space. There is no concept of absolute time or the flow of time, and most importantly there is no arrow of time, it has no directional character: time is isotropic – the same in each direction, forward and backward. The whole process of the discovery of this is described in detail in Pais' book *Subtle is the Lord*:

> Sometime between August 10th and August 16th [1912] it became clear to Einstein that Riemannian Geometry is the correct mathematical tool for what we now call general relativity theory. The impact of this abrupt realisation was to change his outlook on physics and physical theory for the rest of his life. The next three years were the most strenuous period in his scientific career.[21]

Riemannian geometry is of course non-Euclidean, with a positive curvature of space. Therefore the curvature of space due to the presence of mass is the cause of gravitation. It is a geometrical explanation, using non-Euclidean geometry. It is remarkable to think that it took seven years after the special theory of 1905 to come to that discovery. In popular books on Einstein's relativity this can all be described in less than half an hour for adults and even for children, and yet the most famous scientist of the twentieth century took seven years to discover it! The question then arises is it true, is it the final truth about gravitation? The explanation of gravitation as due to the curvature of space of non-Euclidean geometry has momentous consequences for cosmology. It is obvious that if space is curved it must be finite but unbounded. The concept of the possibility of an expansion of the universe and its contraction in the past thus has meaning. Similarly, since space is curved, the universe can have a finite diameter, therefore the concept of multiple universes has meaning.

The years from 1912 to 1915 were spent by Einstein in developing the mathematical formulation of his general theory of relativity. The differential equations used had to reflect the indifference to any particular frame of reference, they had to be invariant under all transformations of the space–time coordinates. For this purpose Einstein used the tensor calculus, which was a generalised vector algebra appropriate for expressing equations of relativity in covariant form. The calculus of tensors was developed by Ricci and Levi-Civita and a special article on it and its application to mathematical physics was published in 1901. Einstein's friend Marcel Grossmann introduced him to the tensor calculus and collaborated with him in its application to general relativity. Tensors are generalisations of vectors, which are tensors of Rank 1, while scalars are tensors of Rank 0. The original concepts of vectors and scalars were first used by Hamilton. Those mathematicians familiar with Hamilton's work were prominent in developing the mathematics of relativity. An excellent example of this is the work of J.L. Synge, the co-editor with A.W. Conway of Volume 1 of Hamilton's *Mathematical Papers*. He has written a book on special relativity, another on general relativity and a book on tensor calculus with A. Schild. The concept of invariance used in general relativity includes invariance with respect to time, i.e. once again excluding any flow of time or arrow of time from the whole theory.

My theory of space–time or more correctly time–space used spin as the fundamental motion. The mathematical formulation of this time–space was Hamilton's quaternions. The quaternion – a quadruple algebra – has four numbers, of which the first one is a scalar and the remaining three are vectors i, j, k, whose square is -1 and which are the axes of spin – i.e. they give the direction of the axes of spin. The first symbol – the scalar – is for time. Time is not the fourth dimension of space – it is the first symbol and is extra-spatial. The scalar number for time can have two possibilities: it can extend to minus infinity or it can have a beginning. If time is infinite in the past it is symmetrical, isotropic, it has no arrow. But if it had a beginning, time would be asymmetrical, have an arrow, and be anisotropic – i.e. not the same in each direction. If we assume that time has a beginning and an arrow we can apply this concept to the problem of gravitational attraction.

In Chapter XIX ('The Gravitational Field') of his book *Relativity: The Special and General Theory*, Einstein writes: 'If we pick up a stone and then let it go, why does it fall to the ground? The usual answer to this question is: Because it is attracted by the Earth.' The earth produces in its surroundings a gravitational field which acts on the stone and produces its motion of fall. Bodies under the influence of gravitation receive an acceleration which does not depend on the material or the physical state of the body. If the incident of dropping the stone is put on videotape and then played backwards, in effect reversing the flow of time, the stone rises from the ground back to one's hand. If it is played forwards, i.e. with the forward flow of time, the stone falls or is attracted to the ground. This can be interpreted as an explanation of gravitation: it is due to the flow of time in one direction – i.e. time with an arrow, asymmetric time. The explanation of gravitation is therefore changed from that of a phenomenon that is spatial and non-Euclidean geometrical to one that is an effect of time which is asymmetrical and has an arrow. For this occurrence time must have a beginning: there must be an absolute scale of time starting at zero. This theory has several important consequences. The space of events remains Euclidean and can be considered infinite in extension; therefore there is only one universe, and multiple universes have no meaning. As the universe could be infinite in extent the expansion of the universe has no meaning – the universe is as large as the mind can conceive. As time which has a beginning is irreversible, gravitation is always attractive, and a force or motion of repulsion is impossible.

The concept of only one universe is particularly important from a philosophical point of view. One can think of a logical universe existing in Euclidean space and in time which is flowing, i.e. asymmetrical and with an arrow. These are all consequences of a beginning of time, an absolute scale of time. If the universe is non-Euclidean, then the possibility of multiple universes is conceivable. The very special problem for gravitation is its unification with quantum theory. Einstein called it a unified field theory, but all his attempts to solve this final problem were not a success and no one else has succeeded yet. The problem is applying quantum theory to gravitation – a theory of quantum gravity. I believe the explanation of gravity as a consequence of an arrow of time will assist in solving this problem.

5 Quantum theory

It is accepted that quantum theory is more fundamental than gravitation theory. Some of the greatest names in physics are responsible for its development and mathematical formulation. These include Planck, Einstein, Bohr, de Broglie, Heisenberg, Schrödinger and Paul Dirac; all these founders of quantum theory were present at the fifth Solway conference in October 1927.

The following is a list of the principal facts and phenomena of quantum theory:

1 Energy available at atomic level is in fixed packets or quanta.
2 There is a particle and wave duality.
3 It includes Heisenberg's uncertainty principle.
4 It involves the Copenhagen interpretation of Heisenberg's uncertainty principle.
5 It involves the existence of the motion of spin – i.e. intrinsic angular momentum – in atomic particles, e.g. the electron.
6 It includes non-locality.
7 The mathematical formulation used includes matrix mechanics and wave mechanics and use of non-commutative algebra.
8 There is no arrow of time.
9 There is constancy of the speed of light.
10 Change is continuous in classical mechanics and relativity; change is discontinuous in quantum theory.

The first real break with classical physics came in 1900 with Max Planck's discovery of the fixed packets of energy involved in electromagnetic radiation:

$$E = h\nu$$

Here, ν is the frequency of the radiation and h is Planck's constant whose value is 6.63×10^{-34} Joule-seconds. Bohr's theory of the atom was published in 1913 to explain the line spectrum of hydrogen. He assumed that a single electron of mass m travelled in a circular orbit of radius r around a positively charged nucleus.

The orbital angular momentum of the electron would be mvr. Bohr proposed that electrons could only occupy orbits in which this angular momentum had certain fixed values, e.g. $h/2\pi$, $2h/2\pi$, $3h/2\pi$, $nh/2\pi$, where h is Planck's constant. The orbital angular momentum is quantified, i.e. can only have certain values, each of which is a multiple of n. Each value of n is associated with an orbit of different radius and when the atom emits or absorbs radiation of frequency ν the electron jumps from one orbit to another; the energy emitted or absorbed at each jump is equal to $h\nu$. It is impossible to apply these ideas of discontinuity, the quantum jumps, to the theory of gravitation. The earth in its orbit around the sun cannot be conceived as jumping from one orbit to another. But if there was some change in the size of the orbit, i.e. its diameter with the progression of time, then the orbit would be different with time. If the orbit was in a very fine spiral it would change continuously, i.e. no jumps would be involved. The same process of change could apply to the atom as well as to the motion of the earth in its orbit around the sun. In particle and wave duality entities such as electrons and photons behave both as if they were particles and also as if they were waves. Hamilton's papers on *On a General Method in Dynamics* appeared in 1834.

His theory of dynamics was so generalised that the laws of light and moving particles could be expressed in the same form. Schrödinger used this discovery of Hamilton's in his theory of wave mechanisms in 1926. He expressed his opinion on Hamilton's work:

> The modern development of physics is constantly enhancing Hamilton's name. His famous analogy between optics and mechanics virtually anticipated wave mechanics, which did not have much to add to his ideas and only had to take them seriously ... If you wish to apply modern theory to any particular problem, you must start putting the problem in *Hamiltonian form*.[22]

Heisenberg's uncertainty principle was discovered in 1927. This asserts that certain pairs of observables (such as position and momentum or time and energy) cannot be known to a greater degree of accuracy than is specified by a limit expressed in terms of Planck's constant. This is a fundamental indeterminism in quantum physics and was accepted as a fact of nature by Bohr. Einstein never accepted this indeterminism in quantum physics with its apparent rejection of causality. His idea was expressed in the famous dictum 'God does not play dice', i.e. rejecting the chance element in quantum theory. It is impossible to apply this concept to gravitation. How could there be indeterminism in the motion of the planets? Bohr's explanation – the Copenhagen interpretation – is that the act of measurement of atomic particles must be taken into consideration. According to this interpretation, the subatomic particles are so minute that the act of measurement interferes with the result. If the particles or objects to be measured are large, there is no indeterminism or imprecision. Roger Penrose comments on this problem in his book *The Emperor's New Mind*: 'We know that at the level of cricket balls, it is classical physics. Somewhere in between, I would maintain, we need to understand the new law, in order to see how the quantum world merges with the classical.' Penrose says that the resolution of the puzzles of quantum theory must lie in our finding an improved theory. At the level of the motion of the planets any effect of measurement is totally absent, and there is no indeterminism or uncertainty. It would seem that quantum theory cannot be applied to gravitation theory.

Paul Dirac in his classic book on quantum mechanics explains the same point of view very clearly:

> The value of the classical analogy in the development of quantum mechanics depends on the fact that classical mechanics provides a valid description of dynamical systems under certain conditions, when the particles and bodies composing the systems are sufficiently massive for the disturbance accompanying an observation to be negligible. Classical mechanics must therefore be a limiting case of quantum mechanics.[23]

It is quite obvious that – as has already been mentioned – quantum mechanics cannot be applied to the motion of the planets if the Copenhagen interpretation is maintained. The only way to solve the problem and allow quantum theory to be applied to gravitation is to find another explanation of the uncertainty and indeterminism in quantum mechanics by some form of hidden variable.

The phenomenon of spin

We have already encountered the phenomenon of spin and based our theory of time–space on spin and not on the motion of translation. In pre-Copernican cosmology the earth was the centre of the universe and had no motion. Since the Copernican Revolution of 1543 the earth has had two motions, one of translation in its orbit around the sun and the other the rotation or spin around its axis each day. Almost all scientific study of the solar system was concentrated on the orbital motions of the various planets, and the study of the earth's spin was neglected until more recent times. The discovery of the spin of atomic particles, e.g. the electrons and photons, in some way provides a link between gravitation theory, which includes the two motions of translation and spin, and the spin of quantum theory. Of the two types of motion it could be maintained that the motion of spin – intrinsic angular momentum – is the more fundamental. The motion of translation is relative, whereas the motion of spin is absolute, as shown by Foucault's pendulum and the use of gyroscopes. I have already based the theory of time–space on the motion of spin, using Hamilton's quaternions as its mathematical formulation.

Non-locality

The phenomenon of non-locality is one of the strangest and most mysterious in quantum mechanics. John Barrow has given an excellent and clear account of the phenomenon:

> The new facet of the laws of Nature this experiment reveals is that the inevitable effect of the act of observation can be non-local; that is, it has effects upon events that are far away, in the sense of being outside the influence of light signals, and hence of any means of information transfer. The measurement of the spin of the first photon instantaneously brings into being the spin value of the second one. This seems completely contrary to common sense. We recall that one of the reasons why Newton's original theory of gravitation was unsatisfactory was because it demanded instantaneous effects arising on things here as a result of events far away. We should add that this non-local effect has been demonstrated in a series of real EPR experiments by the French physicist Alain Aspect and his colleagues in 1982. They in effect changed the initial spin state every ten billionth of a second, and in the meantime made measurements on the equal and opposite spins of the decay products when they were separated by four times the distance that light could travel in the time interval since the initial spin was altered.[24]

A local explanation of the phenomenon is not acceptable: it must be non-local, as Barrow says. If your view of reality is the right one, then it must be a non-local one. If 'hidden variables' did really exist, then faster-than-light signalling would be required.

The mathematics of quantum theory

The most important type of mathematics used in quantum theory is non-commutative algebra. This is beautifully expressed by Paul Dirac in his *Principles of Quantum Mechanics*:

> We now have a complete algebraic scheme involving three kinds of quantities, bra Vectors, ket Vectors and linear operators. They can be multiplied together in the various ways discussed above, and the associative and the distributive axioms of multiplication always hold, but the commutative axiom of multiplication does not hold.[25]

This is non-commutative algebra, which of course was first discovered by Hamilton in 1843 in his quaternions. This discovery was only made after more than ten years of the intense thought and effort required to make such a radical break with all previous algebra, where the commutative law was axiomatic. The matrix mechanics used by Heisenberg is also non-commutative. The fundamental formula expressing the non-commutative multiplication is:

$$qp - pq = ih/2\pi$$

In classical mechanics:

$$qp = pq$$
or $$qp - pq = 0$$

The whole concept of non-commutative algebra seems very strange and almost contradictory. The very word 'equation' means that two expressions are equal, yet by changing the order of multiplication they are no longer equal. My granddaughter, who was aged 13 at the time, made a useful contribution to the linguistic analysis of the algebra used in quantum mechanics. I gave her my copy of Dirac's classical work on the subject and asked her to count the number of times that the terms 'commute', 'commutability' and 'anti-commute', etc. occurred. She gave the total as 278. This is the clearest example of the fundamental importance of the concept. She also counted the number of times 'Hamiltonian' was used and gave the total as 107, which again is the clearest evidence of the importance of Hamilton's dynamics in quantum theory.

E.T. Whittaker has a very valuable paper on non-commutative algebra. It was first given in an address to the Royal Society of Edinburgh when he was its President, on 25 October 1943. The title is 'The New Algebras and Their Significance For Physics and Philosophy'. Whittaker began by referring to Hamilton's discovery of quaternions almost exactly a hundred years before, on 16 October 1843. The quaternion calculus was the prototype of all of the symbolisms which disobey the rules of ordinary algebra, i.e. non-commutative multiplication. Whittaker gives an interesting interpretation of the new algebra:

> This example suggests that, for the purpose of atomic physics, we should investigate the properties of an algebra whose symbols stand for operations like that last described, in which a set of numbers is transformed into another set of numbers, by means of linear equations. Such an algebra was in fact introduced by Cayley not long after the discovery of quaternions; it is called matrix algebra, and it has been shown to be capable of representing quantistic phenomena and furnishing predictions regarding them. Non-commutative algebra is, in fact, the symbolism appropriate to things that cannot be measured exactly.[26]

That which 'cannot be measured exactly' is an imprecision. Using the concept of imprecision instead of indeterminism suggests the possibility of exact precision being attainable. The imprecision is of course fixed and immovable with respect to time. It suggests the possibility of a hidden variable which could eliminate the imprecision and produce a change with the progression of time.

Time and quantum theory

On this problem it is useful to refer to a most important book published recently (1995), namely Paul Davies' *About Time*, with the subtitle, 'Einstein's Unfinished Revolution'. Chapter 7 is entitled 'Quantum Time' and has a section entitled 'Time Vanishes':

> The core difficulty with quantum time harks back to the very notion of Einstein's time; there is no absolute and universal time, my time and your time are likely to be different, and neither is 'Right' or 'Wrong'; they are all equally acceptable. Viewed in terms of four-dimensional space-time, different choices of time correspond to different ways of slicing or decomposing space-time into sections.[27]

and again:

> It must be said that many leading physicists are profoundly unhappy with the foregoing conclusion, and have laboured hard to unearth some 'true' intrinsic time buried obscurely within the mathematics of general relativity. They hope that some ingenious and subtle combination of quantities describing the geometry of

space-time may be revealed to possess the qualities one might expect for a universal measurement of time, and that henceforth this universal time might serve as a genuine 'background' for the measurement of change. So far, however, there is no evidence that such intrinsic time exists.[28]

I have already provided a theory of universal or absolute time based on the motion of spin (intrinsic angular momentum). The mathematical formulation for time–space is Hamilton's quaternions – a quadruple algebra. The first symbol – a scalar – is for time, while the other three represent the three axes of a body subject to spin, i, j, k. The scalar part for time is represented by a horizontal line which is assumed to have a beginning at zero. Because time has a beginning it is asymmetric, has an arrow and is anisotropic. We now have an absolute time scale, a space which is Euclidean and gravitation as a consequence of the arrow of time. The explanation of gravitation is transferred from non-Euclidean geometry to time which has an arrow and which is asymmetric and anisotropic, which is exactly what is required for all change in biology and human experience and in physics. There is no longer a mismatch between physical time and psychological time and the time in biology.

We will show again the five laws of nature for gravitation theory and quantum theory in two columns:

The laws of nature	
Gravitation theory	**Quantum theory**
1 The conservation laws	The conservation laws
2 Symmetry	Symmetry
3 Equations of motion commute	Equations of motion do not commute
4 Speed of light constant	Speed of light constant
5 Uniformity of nature	Uniformity of nature

As already explained these are not really five different laws, since they are all expressing the same fundamental phenomenon, the invariance of nature with respect to time – i.e. the absence of an arrow of time, Time is symmetric or, more properly, isotropic – the same in each direction. All the laws are the same in either theory, except for number 3. In gravitation theory – i.e. general relativity – the equations of motion are equal, they commute. In quantum theory the equations of motion are not equal, they do not commute. These are contradictory concepts and the unification of the two theories is logically impossible.

We will give the type of mathematics used in each theory:

Mathematics		
	General relativity **Gravitation theory**	**Quantum theory**
Geometry	Non-Euclidean Four-dimensional	Hilbert-space n-dimensional
Algebra	Commutative	Non-commutative

It is obvious that the mathematics in each theory are completely different. It therefore seems impossible to unify the two theories. The n-dimensional space of quantum theory is a mathematical fiction – it is a way of expressing the statistical character of quantum mechanics. The atoms in a living body cannot be in n-dimensions – that has no meaning. The natural world or living world exists in the three dimensions of space.

The constancy of the speed of light is a fundamental factor in establishing the invariance of the laws of nature. In the special theory of relativity gravitation is totally absent. This is an unreal and unnatural state of affairs – an absence of gravitation has no meaning. Gravitation is a consequence of the flow of time in one direction, resulting in asymmetric time, anisotropic time. Then the possibility of a change in the speed of light with the progression of time must be considered. The change could be over long periods of time, e.g. millions of years. In 1975 the General Conference of Weights and Measures (CGPM) estimated the speed of light at 299,792,458 metres per second with an uncertainty of $\pm 4 \times 10^{-9}$. In 1983 the same conference gave the same value for the speed of light but without any uncertainty. The value is now taken to be exact. Thus the speed of light ceased to be a measurable constant, and no further determinations of its value will be made. At the end of the last century, physicists were convinced that no further important discoveries would be made in their science, and that all that was required was to add a few figures to give a more accurate value to the constants of physics. However, since 1983 it has been decided that the speed of light as determined in that year is exact to the nearest metre. This seems unreasonable. Is the speed of light exactly the same in 500 million years' time and 500 million years in the past? It seems more logical, especially if time has an arrow and is anisotropic, i.e. is not the same in each direction, that the speed of light should change with time. Paul Dirac had considered that the gravitation constant was changing with time. What is required is the application of an arrow of time to gravitation theory and quantum theory.

We must now consider what effect an arrow of time, i.e. anisotropic time, would have on the two kinds of motion in nature, the translatory motion of the planets in orbit around the sun – orbital angular momentum – and the motion of spin – intrinsic angular momentum. If there is no arrow of time the motion of the planets is in an ellipse which is closed. The rotation in orbit is the same to the left and the right; it is the same in each direction, i.e. the motion is isotropic. If there was an arrow of time, i.e. anisotropic time, then the rotation would not be the same in each direction, left and right would be different, and the ellipse would be open. The only way this can occur is for the motion, the rotation, to be in a fine spiral. We must next consider the effect of an arrow of time on the motion of spin, or intrinsic angular momentum. If there is no arrow of time the rate of spin would be constant – uniform. In pre-Copernican cosmology the rotation of the celestial sphere was considered absolutely constant and uniform. After the Copernican Revolution the rotation was transferred to the spin of the earth on its axis. Again, the rate of spin was assumed to be perfectly constant. This motion was used by astronomers for the measurement of sidereal time, and it was the most perfect measure of time until as late as 1934. But with the development of very accurate clocks, such as quartz crystal clocks and later with atomic clocks, it was shown that the spin of the earth is not uniform (a fact known to astronomers even before the development of accurate clocks). There were discrepancies in the mean motion of the moon, a phenomenon most clearly observed in the moon due to the rapidity of its motion. There were also discrepancies in the observed motions of the planets in the solar system in proportion to the magnitude of their respective mean motions. These researches led to the adoption of ephemeris time in 1960 and later of dynamical time in 1984. This has consequently led to the adoption of leap seconds at a rate of about one per year. The rate of the spin of the earth on its axis is slowing down at a rate of about 1 second per year of 31.5 million seconds. When Einstein developed the theory of general relativity in 1915–16 he looked for some discrepancy in Newtonian celestial mechanics and found one in the precession of the perihelion of the planet Mercury. His new theory was able to account for the observed discrepancy. The phenomenon of the non-uniform spin of the earth, a minute deviation from uniformity, appears to be very fundamental. The spin is not the same in each direction: left-hand spin is slightly different from right-hand spin – i.e. the spin is anisotropic. It could represent a deviation from the conservation of intrinsic angular momentum. That would correlate with an arrow of time or anisotropic time.

To enable gravitation theory and quantum theory to be unified some fundamental change is required in quantum theory. In gravitation theory the motion of the planets is continuous, but quantum theory involves discontinuous change, with the electrons jumping from orbit to orbit – the 'damned jumps' as Schrödinger called them. What is required is a change of electrons from one orbit to the next over very long periods of time, e.g. millions of years. With this atomic structure would change with the progression of time. This change could take place if the speed of light also changed with time. There would obviously then be a difference in structure between the past and the future. This would have special consequences for cosmology, as will be described in the next section.

6 Cosmology – the Big Bang and the expansion of the universe

Cosmology is the study of the universe as a whole. It was only after Einstein's theory of general relativity of 1915–16 that it became a standard branch of physical science. Stephen Hawking in a recent lecture on quantum cosmology remarked that it used to be considered a pseudo-science:

> There were two reasons for this. The first was that there was an almost total absence of reliable observations. Indeed, until the 1920's about the only important cosmological observation was that the sky at night is dark.[29]

Hawking said that there is a second, more serious objection against regarding cosmology as a science:

> Cosmology cannot predict anything about the universe unless it makes some assumption about the initial conditions.[29]

I would have thought that the rotation of the celestial sphere as perceived by early astronomers was a cosmological phenomenon, but since the Copernican Revolution that rotation has been transferred to the spin of the earth on its axis. As already mentioned, E.T. Whittaker's address as President of the Royal Society of Edinburgh on 23 October 1944 was entitled 'Spin in the Universe'. In it, Whittaker asks what is the cosmological significance of rotation and spin. He says that rotation is a universal phenomenon. The earth and all the other members of the solar system rotate on their axes, and of course spin is fundamental in quantum theory. The phenomenon of spin is more fundamental than the motion of translation.

One can predicate that the cosmos – the universe – exists in space and time. That leads at once to the problem of the geometry of space and the age of the universe – or eternity of the universe if time had no beginning. Einstein's special theory of relativity of 1905 is based on the uniform motion of translation in Euclidean space. Gravitation is completely absent from Einstein's special theory, and it took him seven years, until 1912, to find an explanation for gravitation in non-Euclidean geometry – namely that space is curved due to the presence of mass. It is immediately obvious that the universe is finite but unbounded. If the universe is finite in extension then multiple universes are a possibility, and an infinite number of universes are conceptually possible. As the universe is finite in extension its expansion is a possibility. The spectra of galaxies is shifted to the red. That was interpreted as a Doppler effect due to the recession of the galaxies in the line of sight. This led to Hubble's theory of an expanding universe in 1929. The explanation of the expansion of the red-shift is in effect a spatial one. The galaxies are moving in space and the greater the distance the greater the red-shift of the spectra. Einstein did not accept the expansion of the universe. He regretted the introduction of the cosmological constant to maintain a static universe, calling it 'the biggest blunder of my life'. The steady-state theory of the universe was developed by Bondi, Gold and Hoyle in 1948, and maintained that the universe has always existed in a steady state from all eternity and therefore had no beginning. Matter was continually created to balance the expansion of the universe. This theory was replaced by the Big Bang theory in 1965 as the latter gave a satisfactory explanation of the microwave background radiation. According to this theory, the universe originated at a finite time in the past when the temperature was infinite. The age of the universe commonly given is 15,000 million years. In October 1994 sensational new results from the Hubble Space Telescope gave an age of the universe of only eight billion years instead of the standard 15 billion years. It is known that some stars and galaxies are older than recent estimates of the age of the universe, which is an impossibility. The Big Bang theory and the expansion of the universe give an age of the universe. However, there is no law of physics which can give an age of the universe, and the laws of physics break down at singularities, i.e. the beginning of the universe. Stephen Hawking has a very important comment on this problem:

If the laws of physics break down at singularities, these could break down anywhere. The only way to have a scientific theory is if the laws of physics hold everywhere, including at the beginning of the universe. One can regard this as a triumph for the principles of democracy. Why should the beginning of the universe be exempt from the laws that apply at other points?[30]

The answer to this important problem is very clear to me. The laws of physics cannot give an age of the universe but they break down at the beginning because all the laws are invariant with respect to time. They assume that time is infinite in the past. The time of the laws of physics is symmetrical; it has no arrow, or, more properly, the time in physics is isotropic, the same in each direction. There is no essential change in nature with the progression of time – there is invariance with respect to time.

I have developed a theory of the physical universe, a theory of space–time or, more correctly, time–space. It is based on the motion of spin and not on the motion of translation. The motion of spin has two special characteristics. The first is that the motion is absolute, not relative as for translatory motion. This is proved by Foucault's pendulum and is specially commented on by E.T. Whittaker in his paper 'Spin in the Universe'. The second special phenomenon of spin is that it has two and only two directions, right-handed and left-handed. The mathematical formulation for spin or intrinsic angular momentum is Hamilton's quaternions – a quadruple algebra:

$$a + ib + jc + kd$$

It has two parts: a is the scalar part which represents time, while the vector part is $ib + jc + kd$, which represents space.

In the quaternion, i, j, k are the axes of spin, they are vectors whose squares are all $= -1$. The vectors are not coordinates because they do not give the position of the body in space, since a body subject to spin does not change its position. The scalar part is a real number. Hamilton thought of the numbers as lying on a scale from + infinity to – infinity. If the scale extends to infinity in the past, the time which it represents has no arrow. If it is assumed that time had a beginning then it has an arrow, it is asymmetrical or in the most precise language it is anisotropic, i.e. not the same in each direction. As already described this time which has an arrow is the cause of gravitation. The explanation of gravitation has thus been transferred from one based on space – i.e. a geometric explanation due to the curvature of space provided by non-Euclidean geometry. Since the explanation of gravitation is now that it is a consequence of the flow of time in one direction, i.e. of an arrow of time, there is no need for the curvature of space – space can remain Euclidean and infinite in extent. All the phenomena associated with spin such as precession can occur in Euclidean space.

Another explanation of the red-shift of the galactic spectra is thus required. The standard explanation is a spatial one, namely that the galaxies are receding due to the expansion of the universe. The new explanation of the red-shift which I am proposing is based on change due to the progression of time. I have already suggested that there could be a change in the speed of light with time. If the speed of light is increased in the past, the frequency is decreased giving a shift to the red – the effect is thus due to the progression of time alone. For example, Galaxy A is distant 500 million light years and the red-shift is 50 angstrom units. But 500 million years ago the light from the earth and the sun was also shifted the same amount to the red. At the present time the light on Galaxy A shows no shift. In the future, if the speed of light is decreasing the frequency is increasing, with a shift of the light to the blue for Galaxy A and the sun. All these changes require an absolute scale of time – cosmic time – which is provided by the theory of time–space based on the motion of spin. The changes in the spectra of all galaxies and stars in the universe take place at the same cosmic time or epoch. Therefore the concept of simultaneity for the whole universe is restored. These theories about the effects of change in the speed of light are described in my book *The Logical Universe: The Real Universe* with a diagram showing the simultaneous changes in spectra with time.[31]

The biggest change in this theory of cosmology is the introduction of an arrow of time – time which is asymmetric and anisotropic. This is used as the explanation for gravitation. In consequence there is no need for non-Euclidean geometry, i.e. curved space, as an explanation for the phenomenon of gravitation. Therefore Euclidean space can be retained as the geometry of the universe, with immense advantages. The universe with the flat space of

Euclidean geometry can be infinite in extent. There is no meaning to an expansion of the universe and no need for a Big Bang. With the assumption of time with a beginning, the concept of absolute time is restored.

The concept of a change in the speed of light, increased in the past and decreased in the future, provides an explanation for the red-shift of the galactic spectra. The explanation is based on the change produced with the progression of time. If the speed of light is increasing in the past, the frequency is decreasing, with a shift of light to red. If the speed of light reached a limit of infinity at the beginning of time, this would provide the initial condition of the universe, with a temperature reducing to absolute zero at the beginning. With the progression of time temperature is increasing – the opposite effect to the second law of thermodynamics. In this whole theory everything depends on time having a beginning. This is taken as an assumption for the purposes of the present discussion: the explanation for it will be provided later.

7 The philosophy of science – especially the philosophy of mathematics and its applications to nature

The philosophy of science includes of course the philosophy of mathematics. Many scientists are very much opposed to the importance and value of the philosophy of science. They are convinced that it is of no use for the working scientist and has not helped their discoveries in any way. Lewis Wolpert has expressed very definite opinions on this problem in his book *The Unnatural Nature of Science*:

> I do however strongly deny the relevance of these problems to science. It is essential not to mix up the philosophers' problems in dealing with truth, rationality and reality with the success or otherwise of science. My own position, philosophically, is that of a common sense realist. I believe there is an external world which can be studied. I know that philosophically my position may be indefensible but – and this is crucial – holding my position will have made not one iota of difference to the nature of scientific investigation or scientific theories. It is irrelevant.[32]

and again:

> Even distinguished philosophers of science like Hilary Putnam recognise the failure of philosophy to help understand the nature of science.[33]

Wolpert is maintaining that philosophy is of no use or value to the working scientist, that it has been of no help in leading to new discoveries. He is quite correct in these opinions and has made a very valuable contribution to the problem of the irrelevance of philosophy to the working scientist.

The distinguished American scientist and Nobel prizewinner Steven Weinberg has expressed very similar opinions in his book *Dreams of a Final Theory*. The whole of Chapter 7 of the book is on this issue, as shown by the title 'Against Philosophy':

> I am not alone in this, I know of *no one* who has participated actively in the advance of physics in the post war period whose research has been significantly helped by the work of philosophers. I raised in the previous chapter the problem of what Wigner calls the 'Unreasonable Effectiveness' of mathematics; here I want to take up another equally puzzling phenomenon, the unreasonable ineffectiveness of philosophy.[34]

These two scientists have made a clear case for the uselessness of philosophy for the working scientist. But this is not the end of the matter. After scientific discoveries are made scientists often comment and write about the philosophical implications of the discoveries which have been made. There are two good examples of this. The first is Sir James Jeans' book *Physics and Philosophy*. In it he makes a most valuable and important comment on mathematics:

> Mathematicians now employ algebras, which they describe as non-commutative, in which pq is not the same thing as qp; these are found to be specially applicable to the sub-atomic world.[35]

and again with further comment:

> But this is not so; pq–qp has one value in quantum mechanics and a different value, namely zero, in the classical mechanics. The real difference is that the value of pq–qp is mentioned explicitly in the quantum mechanics, but not in the classical mechanics, where p and q are tacitly assumed to be of such a nature that pq must be equal to qp.[36]

This is of course an important comment. It means in effect that quantum theory cannot be applied to classical mechanics and celestial mechanics in the orbital motion of the planets. The second example of a scientist commenting on the usefulness of philosophy after scientific discoveries have been made is the book *Physics and Philosophy* by Werner Heisenberg, one of the founders of quantum theory. The book has exactly the same title as Jeans' work. I will give only one quotation from it:

> To begin with, it is important to remember that in natural science we are not interested in the universe as a whole, including ourselves, but we direct our attention to some part of the universe and make that the object of our studies.[37]

It is surprising that such a famous scientist can be so mistaken. The entire area of study of cosmology is the universe as a whole, which exists in space–time. The fact of giving an age to the universe is a predicate of the universe as a whole. Numerous articles and books have been written on the philosophical implications of Einstein's special and general theories of relativity, especially on his theory of space and time.

Another reason why the philosophy of science, especially the philosophy of mathematics, is no use for the working scientist is that it is the wrong philosophy. The standard philosophy of mathematics is axiomatic set theory. But that was no use or help to Einstein in providing the mathematical formulation for his special and general theories of relativity. That was provided by Minkowski and Marcel Grossmann with the use of tensor analysis, a development of vector analysis. The non-commutative algebra used in quantum theory was not provided by the standard philosophy of mathematics.

Logic

For any philosophy of science, especially physics and the philosophy of mathematics, a theory of logic is a fundamental requirement. Three different types of logic can be described:

1 One-value logic
Here a judgement is true of necessity, i.e. an axiom. This is a theory of identity. The judgement has one reference, the True:

Judgement ————————————►True

2 Two-value logic

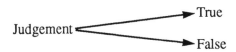

Here the judgement has two references, the True and the False:
The True and the False are two states of affairs, what is the case and what is not the case. This is a theory of difference, called dialectical logic. It can be used to describe Euclidean and non-Euclidean geometry, commutative algebra and non-commutative algebra:

$$ab = ba$$
$$ab \neq ba$$

It is thus a theory of difference or non-identity.
Two-value logic has very valuable application for the description of time

which is symmetrical or asymmetrical, with an arrow or no arrow, isotropic or anisotropic, the same in each direction – i.e. with an identity – or not the same in each direction – i.e. with a difference.

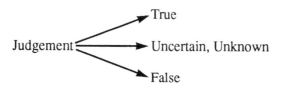

3   Three-value logic

This is analogous to the Scottish law system where the verdict can be either guilty, not guilty or not proven, the last ruling being due to the uncertainty or ignorance of the full facts of the case.

Proof theory requires true premises – which are axioms. With dialectical logic, i.e. two-value logic, there are no axioms. Everything is falsifiable. It can be called a theory of meaning since, as Ayer says, it is only a significant proportion that can be significantly contradicted. A judgement has meaning in the fullest sense only if it can have two references, the True and the False, what is the case and what is not the case. In Abelard's language *Sic et non* – yes *and* no, not yes *or* no. There is both a state of affairs corresponding to yes and a state of affairs corresponding to no.

Reality

A theory of logic must be linked with a theory of reality – a theory of being. I conceive the universe as one reality, one Being existing in time and space. The basic reality is not then of individuals. Living beings and human beings are individuals but the material physical universe is considered as only one reality. The being of the cosmos, the universe as a whole, should be spelt with a capital letter: 'Being'. The word used to describe living beings and human beings is 'being' without the capital letter. As the universe – the cosmos – is considered as one reality the ultimate theory about it must be coherent, i.e. form a single unified theory. There are separate bodies in the universe, e.g. stars and planets. Their structure and motion are fundamental problems. The motion of bodies are of two kinds:

a)   translation
b)   spin, or intrinsic angular momentum.

There is no philosophy of physics without mathematics. Therefore some philosophy of mathematics is absolutely essential for an understanding of the natural world. But there is still no adequate philosophy of mathematics available. John Barrow in his book *Pi in the Sky* has important comments on this problem. In the preface he states:

> Philosophy of mathematics is a steadily evolving subject; but that part of it that deals with the nature of mathematics is stuck in a time warp. The philosophy of mathematics has hardly progressed at all when compared with the development of philosophy or of mathematics. Now is the time to rejuvenate a study of the meaning of mathematics amongst philosophers.[38]

and again on the second from last page of the book:

> all our surest statements about the nature of the world are mathematical statements, yet we do not know what mathematics 'is'; we know neither why it works nor where it works; if it fails or how it fails.[39]

The standard theory of mathematics, e.g. axiomatic set theory, is the foundation of mathematics on axioms. This was specially emphasised by David Hilbert. As physics must be based on mathematics it follows logically that physics must be based on axioms. This point of view was expressed by Hilbert at the International Congress of Mathematics in Paris in 1900. He gave a list of 23 problems in mathematics for future research. Number six was to axiomatise mathematical physics. Axioms are judgements with only one reference, the True – an 'identity' in Wittgenstein's language, a tautology. Axioms are the basis of proof theory. You require true premises – i.e. premises that are true of necessity. If a judgement has two references – the True and the False – it is a theory of meaning. All judgements are falsifiable: this is binary logic, or dialectical logic. It can be used to include commutative and non-commutative algebra. For my book *The Logical Universe: The Real Universe*, published in 1994, I wrote a very brief summary of the central ideas contained in the book. This was not published in the book itself, but was only used in the advertising literature. The following is part of it:

> The central concept of the system of philosophy developed in the book is that of meaning. This is applied to logic as a theory of meaning rather than the proof theory of formal logic. Time is asymmetric, that is it has a direction – an arrow. This concept is applied to the laws of nature which have no arrow of time. In the philosophy of mathematics the same emphasis is on meaning using ideas of Sir William Rowan Hamilton on the ordinal character of numbers, the real numbers, measure numbers, the scalar numbers and the extension to vectors.

The fundamental concept of the philosophy of mathematics must be the concept of number. But there are two different concepts of number. We can go back to Husserl, who makes a clear distinction between the two types of numbers. Husserl's *Philosophy of Arithmetic* appeared in 1891, but earlier, in 1887, he wrote an essay 'On The Concept of Number', of which the subtitle is 'Psychological Analysis'. In it Husserl states that common consciousness finds two sorts of numbers: cardinal numbers and ordinal numbers:

> As cardinal numbers refer to sets, so ordinal numbers refer to series . . . However, noted investigators such as W. R. Hamilton, H. Grassmann and L. Kronecker among others have held the natural starting point is the series. In this way they hope to show the superiority of ordinal numbers (or related concepts) in respect to generality.[40]

Number is a multiplicity of units; other words used are plurality, totality, aggregate, collection and set. A little later Husserl refers to Kant and Hamilton:

> We can omit enumeration of all those investigators who, following Kant, based the concept of numbers upon the representation of time. Let us mention here only two famous names. Sir William Rowan Hamilton flatly called algebra 'the science of pure time', as well as 'science of order in progression'. In Germany H. Von Helmholtz, in a philosophical treatise which recently appeared, has published a detailed investigation into the foundation of arithmetic; and into the justification of the application of arithmetic to physical magnitude.[41]

Husserl described very clearly the kinds of numbers – set numbers, cardinal numbers and series numbers, that is ordinal numbers. But he developed his theory of numbers – his philosophy of mathematics – on the wrong category of numbers. The more fundamental numbers are the ordinals, the series numbers. They are also called scalar numbers, the real measure numbers. My whole philosophy of mathematics is based on this type of number, not on set theory. These theories were developed by Sir William Rowan Hamilton as already described. The very word 'scalar' was used by Hamilton – it refers to the scale of numbers from + infinity to – infinity. He also developed the theory of vectors: the word was first used by him. Hamilton developed the theory of complex numbers as ordered pairs of real numbers, a, b. The complex number is also a vector – a directed line in two dimensions. Hamilton developed his quaternions, which were the extension of vectors to three dimensions. The quaternions are a set of four numbers:

$$a + ib + jc + kd$$

Here, a is the scalar part and $ib + jc + kd$ are the vector part. My interpretation of the symbols i, j, k is that they are the axes of a body subject to spin.

174

The first symbol *a* represents time, while *i, j, k* are vectors but not coordinates as already explained. Coordinates give the position of a body in space and its translation in space, but a body subject to spin – e.g. a top or gyroscope – is not moving from place to place. The axis of spin can point in different directions. The vector representing the axis can be called a direction vector. The multiplication of quaternions is non-commutative:

$$ij = +k$$
$$ji = -k$$

+*k* is left-hand spin
−*k* is right-hand spin

As already explained I have used the quaternion algebra as the mathematical formulation of time–space based on the motion of spin – not on translation as in Minkowski's four-dimensional space–time. The latter formulation has no arrow of time, and time is symmetrical. On the other hand, if *a* the scalar part of the quaternion represents time and is assumed to have a beginning, then time is asymmetrical – i.e. it has an arrow, or in more expressive language time is anisotropic, i.e. not the same in each direction. There is no longer a mismatch between the time of human experience and human history and that of living beings – there is the same arrow of time in each. This makes this theory much superior to the special theory of relativity and the mathematical formulation by Minkowski. Simon Altman gives a very clear and useful account of the difference between rotation and spin. By rotation he means a motion of translation:

> Notice the crux of the matter is difference between 'to spin' and 'to rotate'. The latter is a coordinate transformation and thus has no history and no time, whereas to spin an object is a process realised in time, and it thus has a history.[42]

The expression 'coordinate transformation' refers to a motion of translation. With spin there is no translation: the motion is absolute and requires no coordinates or frame of reference to describe the motion. As has already been mentioned several times, spin has the unique property of motion in two and only two directions – right-handed and left-handed. There is thus an exact correlation with time, which also has two and only two directions – forward and backward. If the spin is uniform, it is the same in each direction – i.e. the spin is isotropic. If the spin is not uniform, it is anisotropic – i.e. not the same in each direction. This would correspond to an arrow of time in the motion of spin.

The motion of a planet in orbit around the sun is of course a motion of translation. According to the laws of motion the orbit is closed. The motion is the same in each direction – left-handed and right-handed, i.e. the motion is isotropic. If an arrow of time is applied to this motion of translation then the orbit is not closed but is open to a minute degree, as in a spiral. In that case the motion is anisotropic – i.e. not the same in each direction. The algebra for such a motion must be non-commutative. The equation of motion is anticommuting. Therefore non-commutative algebra in the motion of translation – orbital motion – and the motion of spin is the mathematical representation of an arrow of time, asymmetric time or – in the most correct term – anisotropic time.

The concepts of scalar and vector were developed from pure mathematics by Hamilton, yet these are the very concepts which need to be used in describing physical science. This was especially commented on by James Clerk Maxwell:

> A most important distinction was drawn by Hamilton when he divided the quantities with which he had to do into scalar quantities, which are completely represented by one numerical quantity, and vectors, which require three numerical quantities to define them.[43]

These concepts of scalar and vector are the foundation of mathematical physics. They are essential in all branches of physics. One could even say that the vector – the real number which has direction – is the 'cardinal' number, i.e. the most important number in the philosophy of mathematics.

Summary and indications for the unification of physics

1 The theory of time–space is based on the motion of spin – intrinsic angular momentum – and not on the motion of translation. The motion of spin is absolute – no frame of reference is required. Time is also absolute – i.e. one cosmic time.
2 The mathematical formulation of this time–space is Hamilton's quaternions, in which the first symbol of the quadruple algebra is the scalar part of the quaternion and represents time. It is based on the assumption that this scale of time represented by the scalars or real numbers has a beginning.
3 Time with a beginning has an arrow, it is asymmetric and anisotropic.
4 Gravitation is caused by the progression of time in one direction – the arrow of time – and is not due to the curvature of space as in non-Euclidean geometry.
5 Space is Euclidean – i.e. infinite in extent and flat.
6 The motion of the planets is in a fine spiral – the equations of motion are non-commutative.
7 There is no expansion of universe.
8 There is no Big Bang.
9 Quantum theory states that the speed of light varies with time, being increased in the past and reduced in the future.

10 This explains the red-shift of the galactic spectra.
11 There is a change in atomic structure with time, e.g. a change of electrons from one orbit to another over long periods of time – millions of years. The imprecision and discontinuity in quantum theory is thus removed and absolute precision is restored.
12 The geometry used can be Euclidean.
13 The spin of electrons should be anisotropic to correlate with anisotropic time – i.e. not the same in each direction.
14 The change in the speed of light with time is the hidden variable and is the explanation of non-locality. The change in the speed of light takes place in absolute time – cosmic time. By means of this, the concept of simultaneity for all parts of the universe, even the most distant, is restored.
15 The equations of motion are non-commutative – the symbolic representation of the arrow of time.
16 Summary of mathematics:

	Gravitation theory	Quantum theory
Geometry	Euclidean	Euclidean
Algebra	Non-commutative	Non-commutative
	Anti-commuting	Anti-commuting

17 This requires another Copernican Revolution, in which the concept of absolute motion and absolute time is restored. The motion of spin which is absolute is the most fundamental concept in nature.
18 The beginning of time is an assumption which requires explanation and will be provided in the final section.

8 The relation between science and religion – the existence of a God or no God

We must begin with a brief account of the different sciences. They can be broadly listed as the natural sciences and the human sciences. The human sciences are often called in German *Geisteswissenschaften*, i.e. the mental sciences.
The natural sciences can be separated into three groups:

1 Physics, chemistry, astronomy
2 Biology including evolution
3 The human sciences, or mental sciences

The last group includes history, the study of language, the history of physics, astronomy, psychiatry, mathematics, the history of mathematics, and the study of consciousness.

The religions include Judaism, Islam and Christianity. These all accept the belief in a transcendent God who created the world and all it contains. Therefore there are two realities: God – the Creator – and His creatures. All creatures exist in time, but God is outside time and is essentially timeless. A remarkable example of the conviction of God as the Creator is shown in Moses Maimonides' *Thirteen Principles* of the Jewish faith. Of the thirteen principles or articles of the Jewish faith *nine* explicitly accept God as the Creator. The first one is:

> I believe with perfect faith that the creator, blessed be his name, is the Creator and Guide of everything that has been created, and that he alone has made, does make, and will make all things.[44]

Maimonides (1135–1204) was the leading Jewish philosopher of the Middle Ages and had a profound influence on Christian thought, especially on St Thomas Aquinas.

The importance of the study of the relations between science and theology has been specially emphasised by Pope John Paul II. This is contained in a paper he sent to Fr. Vincent Coyne, SJ, Director of the Vatican Observatory, on the occasion of a conference at Castelgandolfo in September 1987. This was to commemorate the three-hundredth anniversary of the publication of Newton's *Philosophiae Naturalis Principia Mathematica* in 1687. One paragraph gives a good summary of his concern:

> Contemporary developments in science challenge theology far more deeply than did the introduction of Aristotle into Western Europe in the thirteenth century. Yet these developments also offer to theology a potentially important resource. Just as Aristotelian Philosophy, through the ministry of such great scholars as St. Thomas Aquinas, ultimately came to shape some of the most profound expressions of theological doctrine, so can we not hope that the sciences of today, along with all forms of human knowing, may invigorate and inform those parts of the theological enterprise that bear on the relation of nature, humanity and God?[45]

The challenge to theology could not be more serious as many distinguished scientists deny the existence of God, i.e. the existence of a God who is a Creator – a direct contradiction of the belief of Judaism, Islam and Christianity. This is the position of atheism. A good example of this standpoint is Professor Lewis Wolpert. In his book *The Unnatural Nature of Science* he accepts that most scientists have had religious beliefs but he says:

> This presents a problem for scientists who have to reconcile their views with religion or reject it, since, as I will try to show, religion and science are incompatible.[46]

and again with more explicit assertions on the opposition of religion and science:

> This might drive some scientists to arguing that God provides the starting-point, and that God wound up the Universe and set it going. But now the scientist is drawn in the opposite direction, for postulating a God is to postulate a causal mechanism for which there is neither evidence nor any foundation – a postulate that cannot be falsified. A scientist may perhaps believe in God, but he or she cannot use God as an explanation for natural phenomena.[47]

The classic example of the opposition between religion and science is the condemnation of the Copernican theory by the Holy Office in Rome in 1616. Galileo was forbidden to teach or defend it. At the same time Copernicus's book *De Revolutionibus Orbium Coelestium* was put on the Index until it was corrected. The book was first published in 1543, the year of Copernicus's death. In 1633 Galileo was tried by the Inquisition for the book he published attacking Ptolemaic astronomy and was condemned for suspected heresy. He was sentenced to imprisonment, which in effect amounted to house arrest. It is obvious in the light of further scientific advances that the Church made a serious error of judgement in trying to stifle the Copernican movement. This is the most important historical evidence of the conflict between science and religion. In this instance science was proved right and the religious point of view wrong.

Scientists have a special objection to the apparent certainty with which religious people accept their beliefs. Lewis Wolpert has expressed it very clearly: 'Unlike scientists, religion is based on unquestioning certainties.' Herman Bondi in an article in *The Times* has expressed it even more clearly. The article is entitled 'The Arrogance of Certainty':

> What I abhor about revealed religion is its supposed absolute certainty. It is here that I see the real conflict between science and religion.[48]

The certain beliefs of religion are called dogmas. But the word 'dogma' is Greek, it literally means an opinion, i.e. a belief, that can be true or false. The contrary opinion of the true one is a heresy. However, every belief can be falsified – for every dogma there is thus a corresponding heresy. The divinity of Christ is a dogma, but its denial is the Arian heresy. The same interpretation applies to the word 'orthodox', used for orthodox faith or religion. The word *doxa* is Greek and means 'opinion'; 'orthodox' means 'right opinion', so obviously a belief which is not orthodox is not the right or true belief. Therefore every belief or judgement about religion is true or false. This is the use of two-value logic, in which every judgement has two references, the True and the False. This is dialectical logic, which contrasts with axiomatic theory, since an axiom is a judgement with one reference only, the True, it is true of necessity. Axioms are the basis of proof theory, since for proof you require true premises, i.e. true of necessity. The existence of a transcendent God who created the universe is a dogma – i.e. an opinion – the true opinion. Yet the theist's false opinion, that there is no God, is also conceptually possible. If there is no God, the universe is all there is and logically it ought to be eternal. Therefore there are two states of affairs – a God and no God. But for the atheist, who is convinced that there is no God, there is no possibility of the existence of a God who created the world. Atheism is not a dogma, i.e. a belief which is true or false; it is true of necessity, it is an axiom which is not falsifiable.

The fact that religious beliefs are falsifiable – that they are not absolute certainties, but can be true or false – was unwittingly confirmed by Richard Dawkins in a letter to *The Independent* newspaper on 12 August 1993. The letter, headed 'The Contradictory Spirit of Religion', was in response to a leading article a few days before. Dawkins gave several examples of contradictory beliefs, e.g. that there is one God, there are many Gods; Jesus is the Son of God and he is not, etc.

> Children must learn the rudiments of the exciting new *Contradiction Theology*: that all religions are simultaneously true and false, and that this is (don't you feel?) a very positive thing . . .[49]

The whole tone of the letter is one of utter contempt for all religion. But the writer unwittingly made the important point that religious beliefs are not axioms, i.e. true of necessity, but dogmas, i.e. opinions which can be true or false. The convinced atheist who believes that there is no God has no possibility of falsifying that belief. For him it is axiomatic and true of necessity. God's existence is for the atheist inconceivable. St Thomas Aquinas developed five proofs for the existence of God. The first one, which he considered the best, was the proof from motion – whatever is in motion must be put in motion by another, which is God, the prime mover. In modern dynamics – with the law of inertia – no mover is required. Now the problem is transferred to the duration of existence of the universe. Is the universe eternal, with time infinite in the past, or did God create the universe at the beginning? This was a very special problem for St Thomas as Aristotle had explicitly maintained that the universe was eternal. St Thomas accepted that the universe had a beginning from revelation. However, his belief that the world began to exist due to its creation by God is an object of faith but not demonstration or science.

The problem of God's existence is not one of proof but of meaning. For meaning you require a judgement which has two references, the True and the False – two states of affairs, what is the case and what is not the case. For the universe and God's existence the problem is whether time had a beginning or no beginning – was the universe in existence from all eternity or did it have a beginning? For the answer to this problem we must consider again the laws of nature.

Steven Weinberg in his book *Dreams of a Final Theory* has the perfect comment on this problem and its possible solution:

> If there were anything we could discover in nature that would give us some special insight into the handiwork of God, it would have to be the final laws of nature. Knowing these laws, we would have in our possession the book of rules that govern stars and stones and everything else. So it is natural that Stephen Hawking should refer to the laws of nature as 'the mind of God'.[50]

We give a list of the laws of nature again:

1 The conservation laws
2 Symmetry
3 The laws of motion expressed as equations
4 The constancy of the speed of light
5 The uniformity of nature

These laws are valid for gravitation theory but not for quantum theory, in which one law – the third – is different. For quantum theory the laws are:

1 The conservation laws
2 Symmetry
3 The equations of motion are not equal. They do not commute
4 The constancy of the speed of light
5 The uniformity of nature

These are not really five different laws, since they are all expressing the same invariance with respect to time. They are a consequence of time which has no arrow, time which extends to infinity in the past – i.e. time which has no beginning. If time has no beginning, there is no need for God. These are the laws corresponding to God's non-existence. John Macquarrie in his book *Heidegger and Christianity* has a very important reference to the problem of atheism:

> The course [of lectures] for 1925 was entitled *History of the concept of time*, and fills a substantial volume of more than three hundred pages. The work is important for at least two reasons. The first is that it is a significant step towards Heidegger's *magnum opus, Being and Time*, which followed two years later. The second reason is that the course of lectures shows the centrality of the problem of time in Heidegger's philosophy . . . Heidegger sometimes speaks in this way too, for instance he says that phenomenology is 'a pure methodological concept which only specified the *how of the research*'. He holds therefore that such research must be, in a methodological sense, atheistic, in the same sense that the natural sciences are atheistic, that is to say, they do not bring in God as an 'explanation' for anything . . . But must not such an investigation come eventually to the problem of theism versus atheism?[51]

Macquarrie points out that the concluding section of Heidegger's *History of the Concept of Time* was entitled 'The Exposition of Time Itself' but was not actually written. The five laws of nature as given are the laws if there is no God, the laws for atheism. As Lewis Wolpert says – and all atheists assert – religion and science are incompatible; there is a conflict between science and religion, wherein science is right and true and religion is wrong and false. I agree that there is a conflict between science and religion, but considering the laws of nature as listed I say that science is wrong or incomplete and religion is right and true – God created the universe at the beginning of time. The five laws of nature have no arrow of time, i.e. time is isotropic. However, if God created the universe at the beginning of time, then there is an arrow of time, i.e. time is anisotropic. Between 1948 and 1965 the standard theory of cosmology was the steady-state theory of Bondi, Gold and Hoyle. This explicitly required that the universe should be eternal – time had no beginning. But as far as I know no Christian theologian rejected this theory and stated that it contradicted Christian belief. They were all afraid to contradict the scientists and say that the latter were wrong and religion was right. Sir Edmund Whittaker in his book *Space and Spirit* has an important comment on this problem. He refers first to the absolute scale of temperature – the Kelvin scale with absolute zero at –273° Celsius:

Similarly if *absolute time* is measured from the natural origin of time (the creation) it may be that the absolute time will enter into some laws of nature.[52]

St Augustine in his book *The City of God* gives a clear account of creation and time. In Book XI, Chapter VI, the heading is 'That the World and Time Had Both One Beginning, Nor Was the One Before the Other'. One brief quotation expresses his point of view very clearly:

And if the holy and most true scriptures say that 'In the beginning God created heaven and earth', to wit, that there was nothing before then, because this was the beginning which the other should have been if aught had been made before, then verily the world was made with time, and not in time, for that which is made in time, is made both before some time, and after some.[53]

St Thomas Aquinas was faced with particular difficulty over the problem of creation with a beginning of time, because Plato and Aristotle had both accepted the eternity of time and the universe. Aquinas' final conclusion was that we only accept the creation of the universe at a beginning of time from revelation. But it cannot be proved from philosophy, although he was prepared to consider the universe existing from eternity as not logically impossible. Cardinal Joseph Ratzinger has a small book on the Catholic understanding of the study of creation based on the revelation in the Old Testament and the New Testament. The title is *In the Beginning*,[54] which has clear significance for the temporal origin of time and the universe. In notes at the end of the book the author complains of the neglect of the doctrine of creation in some modern works of theology. The Reverend John Polkinghorne has the same comment in a recent book *Science and Christian Belief.* He says that the doctrine of creation receives comparatively little attention in contemporary theology: Hans Kung could write a six-hundred-page account of Christianity for the general reader without creation occurring once in the index.

Several Christian theologians have expressed the opinion that a temporal origin of the universe is not essential for the belief in the creation of the universe by God. They believe that He could have created it from all eternity. The universe could thus be considered as dependent on God for its existence without the need for a beginning in time. I will give only one reference to this point of view. It is by the Reverend John Polkinghorne, who has referred to this theory in many of his books. I will quote from one of the latest of these, the aforementioned *Science and Christian Belief* based on the Gifford lectures for 1993–4:

Of course, the first thing to say about that discourse is that theology is concerned with ontological origin and not with temporal beginning. The idea of creation has no special stake in a datable start to the universe . . . Creation is not something he did fifteen billion years ago, but it is something that he is doing now.[55]

I am convinced that this point of view is in error. There are special advantages in the theory of the universe with a beginning. If time had a beginning it has an arrow, it is asymmetric: in the most perfect language, time is anisotropic. In the present laws of physics as listed earlier it is impossible to provide a unification of physics. In gravitation theory the equations of motion are equal, they commute. In quantum theory the equations are not equal, they require non-commutative algebra for their expression. These are contradictory states of affairs whose unification is impossible.

The theory of time–space which I have developed is based on the motion of spin or intrinsic angular momentum and not on the motion of translation as in the special theory of relativity. The motion of spin does not require any coordinates or frame of reference. The mathematical formulation for this theory of time–space based on the motion of spin is Hamilton's quaternions:

$$s + ia + jb + kc$$

In this formula, s is the scalar part and represents time – it is a real number – whereas $ia + jb + kc$ are the vector part, of which i, j, k represent the three directions of the axis of spin – they are not coordinates but vectors whose squares are all -1. Diagrammatically, s – the scalar part for time – can be represented by a horizontal line. Time has two directions, forward and backward. The backward direction has only two possibilities – time extends to infinity in the past or time has a beginning. If time has no beginning there is no arrow of time. If time had a beginning it would have an arrow, and be anisotropic. The geometry of this time–space is Euclidean and a gravitational field is present and provides for the phenomena of spin such as precession. We have already explained that the curvature of space is not necessary to cause gravitation. There is no expansion of the universe and no Big Bang. I had assumed that time had a beginning but had not provided any explanation for this. From what I have already written it is clear that the explanation of a beginning of time is the creation of the universe by God in the beginning. If the universe was created from eternity time would have no arrow, there would be no explanation for gravitation and the unification of physics would be impossible. Therefore a beginning of time is more important from a scientific point of view. In the present theory of cosmology the Big Bang and the expansion of the universe provides an age for the universe. But this theory is incomplete and inadequate to confirm the age of the cosmos because there is no law of nature which can provide such an age of the universe. An atheist could ask a theist a very fair question: 'If you are so sure that God created the universe at the beginning of time, why can't you calculate the age of the universe from some law of nature?' That is a very good question. The answer should be clear from what has already been explained. There is no law of nature which can be used to calculate the age of the universe because all the laws are invariant with respect to time. There is no arrow of time: time is isotropic, i.e. the same in each direction – all a consequence of no beginning of time. All the laws listed are the laws for if there was no God: they are the laws of atheism. The question immediately arises: what would the laws of nature be if there was a God who created the universe at the beginning of time? The following are the laws of physics if time had no beginning and in consequence no arrow:

1 The conservation laws
2 Symmetry
3 The laws of motion expressed as equations
4 The constancy of the speed of light
5 The uniformity of nature.

We must now see how the laws of nature change by the application of an arrow of time, i.e. time with a beginning. The laws are changed by the application of a negation to all the laws:

1 Deviation from the conservation laws
2 Non-symmetry or asymmetry
3 Laws of motion whose equations are not equal and which do not commute
4 Change in the speed of light with time
5 Non-uniformity of nature.

The first five laws as listed are the laws of nature for if there is no God – i.e. no creation, no beginning of time. Therefore there is a conflict between science and religion. For the theist science is wrong or incomplete and religion is right or true: God created the universe at the beginning of time. In consequence of this time has a beginning: it is on an absolute scale beginning at zero, analogous to the absolute scale of temperature, the Kelvin scale. Time is now with an arrow, i.e. it is asymmetric and anisotropic. For the atheist religion is always wrong and science right. The laws of nature are thus obvious and in no need of proof if there is no God. However, this contradicts the fundamental belief of the Jewish, Moslem and Christian religions.

We must describe the changes in the laws of nature following the application of an arrow of time. Many of the consequences have already been given – they are summarised as follows:

1 Deviation from the conservation laws
There is a deviation from the conservation of orbital angular momentum: the right-hand rotation of planets in orbit is different from the left-hand rotation – the motion is not the same in each direction but is anisotropic. This can occur if the motion is open not closed, i.e. motion in a fine spiral. There is also a deviation from the conservation of intrinsic angular momentum or spin. It is already known that the spin of the earth is not uniform, that there is a loss of 1 second in a year of approximately 31.5 million seconds. There is a deviation from the conservation of energy. Using Einstein's equation $E = MC^2$, it is evident that if the speed of light is increased in the past, the energy is reduced.

2 Non-symmetry or asymmetry
This is a consequence of the arrow of time: the flow of time in one direction causes an asymmetry between the past and the future.

3 The laws of motion
The equations of the laws of motion are no longer equal, they do not commute – non-commutative algebra is required.

4 Change in the speed of light with time
The consequences of this change have already been described. They are a change of energy with the passage of time, and a change in the atomic structure resulting in the shift of spectra to red in distant galaxies. The latter is an explanation of the red-shift due to time, not a spatial explanation as in the Doppler effect. This could also explain Olber's paradox – i.e. the darkness of the night sky. The spectra of light from distant galaxies is shifted to red – the greater the distance, the greater the shift and the less the brightness. It could also explain the phenomenon of non-locality, the hidden variable being the change in the speed of light which is not local but

universal in the universe. The concept of simultaneity for the whole universe with an absolute cosmic time can be retained. These laws of nature with the arrow of time can provide for the initial conditions and give an age of the universe.

5   Non-uniformity of nature
The laws of uniformity of nature depend on the absence of an arrow of time, i.e. there is no essential change in nature as there is no flow of time. With an arrow of time nature is no longer uniform, and there is change with the progression of time.

The application of the arrow of time to quantum theory has a special and specific importance. The list of five laws of nature for gravitation theory also applies to quantum theory with the exception of number 3 – the equations of motion are non-commutative already. As E.T. Whittaker has expressed it, non-commutative algebra is in fact the symbolism appropriate to things that cannot be measured exactly. In other words there is an imprecision in quantum theory: this is of course the indeterminism, the statistical character of the theory. But this imprecision is fixed and invariant with respect to the progression of time. With the application of the arrow of time by means of the change in the speed of light the imprecision changes with time – in effect precision is restored. This results in the change in atomic structure over long periods of time, e.g. millions of years. This also restores the factor of continuity in quantum theory and opens the way to the unification of gravitation theory and quantum theory. The mathematics now used in celestial mechanics will no longer be tensor analysis with its fundamental concept of invariance with respect to time. The mathematics used can be Hamilton's theory of dynamics but with the important difference that the equations must be non-commutative or anti-commuting. This is to express or represent the change with the progression of time: the motion of the planets is anisotropic, not the same in each direction, and right-handed and left-handed in orbital rotation, i.e. motion in a fine spiral.

The last chapter in my book *The Logical Universe: The Real Universe* is on natural theology, on the problem of the existence or non-existence of God from the point of view of reason alone. The central problem of time with no beginning and no arrow and time with a beginning and an arrow is set out in a double column, as shown in the table below.

The two columns show clearly the states of affairs as to whether there is a God or no God. This shows the fundamental importance and use of two-value logic, i.e. dialectical logic. We are not using proof theory which requires true premises, i.e. premises that are true of necessity, or axioms. We are using the theory of meaning – that a judgement has two references: what is the case and what is not the case, what is true and what is false. The first column in the table gives the current standard laws of nature for if there is no God. This is why I say that there is a conflict between science and religion – that science is wrong or incomplete and religion is right or true in maintaining that God created the universe at the beginning of time. The first verse of the Old Testament in Genesis is 'In the beginning God created the heaven and the earth.' The first Vatican Council explains:

> This one true God of his own goodness and 'almighty power', not for increasing his own beatitude, nor for attaining his perfection but in order to manifest this perfection through the benefits which he bestows on creatures, with absolute freedom of counsel 'and from the beginning of time, made out of nothing both orders of creatures the spiritual and the corporeal'.[57]

<table>
<tr><td colspan="2" align="center">**Dialectical logic**</td></tr>
<tr><td>*NO GOD*</td><td>*GOD EXISTS*</td></tr>
<tr><td>Time – no beginning</td><td>Time – a beginning</td></tr>
<tr><td>No arrow of time</td><td>Arrow of time</td></tr>
<tr><td>Conservation laws</td><td>Non-conservation laws</td></tr>
<tr><td>Symmetry</td><td>Non-symmetry</td></tr>
<tr><td>Equations of motion are equal</td><td>Equations of motion are not equal</td></tr>
<tr><td>Uniformity of nature</td><td>Non-uniformity of nature</td></tr>
<tr><td>Mathematics are commutative</td><td>Mathematics are anti-commuting</td></tr>
<tr><td colspan="2" align="center">**Idealistic logic – coherent theory**</td></tr>
<tr><td>Physical theories are not coherent</td><td>Physical theories are coherent – one unified theory</td></tr>
<tr><td>The universe is unlogical</td><td>The universe is logical</td></tr>
<tr><td>THE FALSE</td><td>THE TRUE[56]</td></tr>
</table>

The creation of the universe at the beginning of time is a dogma of the Catholic Church. As has already been explained, 'dogma' means an opinion, i.e. the opposite or denial of the dogma is possible. That the universe could have been created from all eternity is thus also a conceptual possibility. For an atheist the non-existence of God as the Creator of the universe is true, and true of necessity; therefore it is an axiom: its denial is impossible, it cannot be falsified.

Professor Lewis Wolpert has important comments on this fundamental problem:

> This might drive some scientists to arguing that God provides the starting-point, and that God wound up the universe and set it going. But now the scientist is driven in the opposite direction, for postulating a God is to postulate a causal mechanism

for which there is neither evidence nor any foundation that cannot be falsified. A scientist may perhaps believe in a God, but he or she cannot use God as an explanation for natural phenomena. He escapes embodied presence and perception since he is not in space and his existence cannot be demonstrated.[58]

Everything in this problem turns on the universe existing in time, and whether it had a beginning. As already explained, Wolpert's assertion that God's existence cannot be falsified is not correct. If there is no God time has no beginning and is symmetrical. All the present standard laws of nature are as they are because there is no God, and time extends in theory to infinity in the past. On the other hand, the atheist's assertion that there is no God is a truth of necessity, and therefore cannot be falsified. He cannot say what would be the case if God created the universe, since for him God's non-existence is axiomatic – true of necessity – and therefore not falsifiable.

Wolpert says that God cannot be used for the explanation of any natural phenomena. This is quite correct for the present state of physics. Therefore scientific atheists are true to their own laws and principles. I have concluded that there is a conflict between science and religion, that science is wrong or, more correctly, incomplete and religion is right and true in the belief that God created the universe at the beginning of time. The present scientific explanation of the beginning of the universe occurring at the Big Bang followed by the expansion of the universe is not adequate, nor of sufficient certainty. It conflicts with the fact that the laws of nature cannot give an age of the universe because they are based on the concept of time being infinite in the past and in consequence time has no arrow and is isotropic, i.e. the same in each direction. The expression used is that the laws of nature 'break down at the singularity', the beginning of the universe as suggested by the Big Bang. As has already been mentioned, Stephen Hawking has a most important and valuable comment on this problem. He says: 'The only way to have a scientific theory is if the laws of physics hold everywhere, including at the beginning of the universe.' The reason they do not hold at the beginning of the universe is the absence of an arrow of time in physics. If God created the universe at the beginning of time there would be an arrow and this could be the explanation of gravitation. Therefore He is the God of gravitation and the God of the arrow of time as a direct consequence of the creation of the universe at a beginning of time. Even so, many Christian scientists do not accept that it is necessary to hold that God created the universe at the beginning of time. They say He could have created it from all eternity. John Polkinghorne is one of the scientists who accept this point of view. In my opinion it is mistaken. If the universe has existed from infinite past time, there is no arrow of time. If time had a beginning it has an arrow and an absolute scale. This results in a change in the laws of physics, which opens the way to a unification of physics.

Professor Peter Atkins of Oxford University is a convinced atheist. The journalist Andrew Grimes has reported Professor Atkins's recent statements about the problem of God's existence:

> 'All religious beliefs,' he declared at this week's conference of the British Association for the Advancement of Science, 'are outmoded and ridiculous. To say that God made the world is simply a more or less sophisticated way of saying that we don't understand how the world originated.' I do not believe in God any more than Professor Atkins does, but I think his arguments give us atheists a bad name![59]

It should be noticed that Atkins does not mention the possibility that God made the world at the beginning of time, which I believe is essential and critical and which I have already explained many times. The scientific explanation of the origin of the universe at the Big Bang followed by the expansion of the universe is not absolutely certain. I have given different explanations based on the effect of an arrow of time in the laws of nature. Professor Atkins wrote a book on creation published in 1981. Since he is an atheist it was rather odd of him to give it the title *The Creation*, because there is obviously no creation if there is no God. The title is an excellent example of irony. Atkins published a second revised and extended edition in 1992 with the title *Creation Revisited* and the subtitle 'The Origin of Space, Time and The Universe'. In the preface he states:

> My aim on the first visit was to argue that the universe can come into existence without intervention and that there is no need to invoke the idea of a supreme being in one of its numerous manifestations.[60]

He is quite correct to say that present-day physics has no need for God. God is not needed to explain anything in physics. But I maintain that there is a conflict between science and religion, that science is wrong or incomplete and religion is right – God created the universe at the beginning of time. The unification of physics with the present laws of nature is impossible because there is no arrow of time. If God created the universe at the beginning of time, then time would have an arrow; time would be anisotropic, with a change in the laws of physics which would result in a unification of physics.

In the second edition of his book *Creation Revisited* Dr Atkins has added a new chapter on mathematics, Chapter 5, called 'Calculating Things'. He has made an important and most valuable contribution to science by emphasising the importance of mathematics for the study of nature:

> One of the deepest problems of nature is the success of mathematics as a language for describing and discovering features of physical reality.[61]

He states that it is not too extravagant to claim that the answer to the question of why mathematics works will be the final answer to all questions of being. He says that no one yet knows why mathematics works. My studies in the philosophy of mathematics will, I hope, provide an answer to the problems. No use has been made of axiomatic set theory: instead I have used the ideas of Sir William Rowan Hamilton on the meaning of mathematics. The emphasis is on the ordinal character of numbers, the real numbers, the scalar numbers and the extension to vectors. The final extension of the number system is to Hamilton's quaternions. Then I realised that quaternion algebra could be the mathematical formulation of a new theory of time–space based on the motion of spin (intrinsic angular momentum), not based on the motion of translation as in the special theory of relativity. This is a return to absolute motion. The first symbol of the quaternion – the scalar part, a real number – represents time. If time had a beginning, it would provide an absolute scale and time would have an arrow. This is a return to absolute time which is asymmetric, i.e. anisotropic – not the same in each direction. There is no mismatch between this time and the time of human experience and living beings. This is superior to Minkowski's mathematical formulation of special relativity. It is another Copernican Revolution – a return to an absolute scale of time flowing in one direction and irreversible.

We now consider Hamilton's famous theory, that algebra is the science of pure time. We can ask the question: is there any difference in the algebra if time had a beginning or no beginning? If time had no beginning it is symmetrical and isotropic and the algebra is commutative. If time had a beginning, it is asymmetrical, anisotropic and the algebra is non-commutative or anti-commuting. There is a difference in the direction of time and the laws of nature according to whether there is a God or no God. This is equivalent to saying that the existence of God has meaning – there are two states of affairs in the laws of physics corresponding to His existence or non-existence.

My final conclusion is: The arrow of time is the key to the universe. This is a consequence of the creation of the universe at the beginning of time. The existence of God has meaning and is the truth – *veritatis splendor* – the splendour of truth.

References

Prolegomenon
Frege – the theory of judgement

1 G. Frege, *Translations from the philosophical writings of Gottlob Frege*, ed. by P. Geach and M. Black (Oxford, Blackwell, 1960), p. 56.
2 E. Husserl, *Logical Investigations*, translated by J.N. Findlay (London, Routledge & Kegan Paul, 1970), Vol. 1, p. 287.
3 Ibid., p. 292.
4 W. and M. Kneale, *The Development of Logic* (Oxford, Clarendon Press, 1962), p. 1.
5 E. Husserl, *Ideas – General Introduction to Pure Phenomenology*, translated by W.R. Boyce Gibson (London, George Allen & Unwin, 1931), p. 176.
6 M. Heidegger, *Being and Time*, translated by J. Macquarrie and E. Robinson (London, SCM Press, 1962), p. 198.
7 Frege, *Translations from philosophical writings*, p. 61.
8 Ibid., p. 62.
9 Ibid., p. 63.
10 G. Ryle, *The Revolution in Philosophy* (London, Macmillan & Co. Ltd, 1960), p. 7.
11 L. Wittgenstein, *Tractatus Logico-Philosophicus*, translated by D.F. Pears and B.F. McGuinness (London, Routledge & Kegan Paul, 1961), section 2.21.
12 Ibid., section 4.023.
13 G.E.M. Anscombe, *An Introduction to Wittgenstein's Tractatus* (London,

Hutchinson University Library, 1959), p. 81.

14 Kneale, *Development of Logic*, pp. 1–2.
15 M. Dummett, *Frege – Philosophy of Mathematics* (London, Duckworth, 1991), p. 170.
16 Ibid., p. 45.
17 I. Kant, *Prolegomena to any Future Metaphysics*, translated by Peter G. Lucas (Manchester, Manchester University Press, 1953), p. 22.
18 Frege, *Translations from philosophical writings*, p.127.
19 Dummett, *Frege – Philosophy of Mathematics*, p. 246.
20 A.J. Ayer, *Language, Truth and Logic* (London, Victor Gollancz, 1946), p. 115.
21 Wittgenstein, *Tractatus Logico-Philosophicus*, section 6.2341.

Chapter 1
Introduction

1 I. Kant, *The Critique of Pure Reason*, translated by J.M.D. Meiklejohn (London, J.M. Dent, 1934), p. 26.
2 E. Husserl, *Ideas I*, translated by W.R. Boyce Gibson (London, George Allen and Unwin, 1931), p. 78.
3 B. Russell, *Introduction to Mathematical Philosophy* (London, George Allen and Unwin, 1919), p. 17.
4 Ibid., p. 96.
5 G. Frege, *The Foundations of Arithmetic*, Eng. trans by J.L. Austin (Oxford, Basil Blackwell, 1953), p. 53.
6 A.J. Ayer, *Language, Truth and Logic* (London, Victor Gollancz, 1946), pp. 86–7.
7 M. Dummett, *Frege – Philosophy of Mathematics* (London, Duckworth, 1991), p. 45.
8 David Bell, *Husserl* (London, Routledge, 1990), p. 81.
9 Ibid., pp. 81–2.

Chapter 2
The concept of number

1 M. Dummett, *Frege – Philosophy of Mathematics*. (London, Duckworth, 1991), p. 246.
2 R. Penrose, *The Emperor's New Mind* (Oxford, Oxford University Press, 1989), p. 86.
3 G. Temple, *100 Years of Mathematics* (London, Duckworth, 1981) p. 3.
4 Dummett, *Frege*, p. 270, fn 13.
5 W.R. Hamilton, *The Mathematical Papers of Sir William Rowan Hamilton* (Cambridge, Cambridge University Press, 1967), Vol. 3, p. 6.
6 Ibid., p. 7.

7 S. O'Donnell, *William Rowan Hamilton* (Dublin, Boole Press, 1983), p. 129.

Chapter 3
Number systems

1 E.T. Whittaker, 'The Sequence of Ideas in the Discovery of Quaternions', *Proceedings of the Royal Irish Academy* (1944), Vol. 50A. No. 6, p. 96.
2 S. O'Donnell, *William Rowan Hamilton* (Dublin, Boole Press, 1983), p. 145.
3 S. Stebbing, *A Modern Introduction to Logic* (London, Methuen, 1946), p. 189 fn 1.
4 A.J. Ayer, *The Central Questions of Philosophy* (London, Penguin Books, 1973), p. 202.
5 O'Donnell, *Hamilton*, p. 151.
6 E.T. Whittaker, 'The Hamiltonian Revival', *The Mathematical Gazette* (1940), Vol. 24. No. 260, p. 153.
7 P.A.M. Dirac, *The Principles of Quantum Mechanics*, 4th edn (Oxford, Clarendon Press, 1958), p. 26.
8 E.T. Whittaker, Reprint from *Year Book of the Royal Society of Edinburgh* (Edinburgh, Oliver and Boyd, 1944), p. 9.
9 M. Dummett, *Frege – Philosophy of Mathematics* (London, Duckworth, 1991), p. 60.

Chapter 4
Algebra – the science of pure time

1 W.R. Hamilton, *The Mathematical Papers of Sir William Rowan Hamilton*, (Cambridge, Cambridge University Press, 1967), Vol. 3. p. 117.
2 Ibid., p. 123.
3 T.L. Hankins, *Sir William Rowan Hamilton* (Baltimore, Johns Hopkins University Press, 1980), p. 271.
4 W.H. Newton-Smith, *The Structure of Time* (London, Routledge and Kegan Paul, 1980), p. 51.
5 S.W. Hawking, *A Brief History of Time* (London, Bantam Press, 1988), p. 152.
6 R. Penrose, *The Emperor's New Mind* (Oxford, Oxford University Press, 1989), p. 302.
7 G.J. Whitrow, *The Natural Philosophy of Time*, (London, Thomas Nelson, 1961), p. 21.
8 St Thomas Aquinas, *Commentary on Aristotle's Physics*, translated by James A. McWilliams S.J. (Washington, Catholic University of America, 1945), p. 81.

9 E. Husserl, *Philosophie der Arithmetic* (Husserliana, The Hague, Nijhoff, 1891), p. 33.
10 G. Frege, *The Foundations of Arithmetic*, translated by J.L. Austin (Oxford, Blackwell, 1884), p. 53.
11 J. Passmore, *A Hundred Years of Philosophy* (London, Duckworth, 1954), pp. 272–3.
12 B. Russell, *Our Knowledge of the External world* (Chicago and London, Open Court Publishing Company, 1914), p. 167.
13 A.J. Ayer, *Language, Truth and Logic* (London, Gollancz, 1946), p. 115.
14 G. Ryle, *The Revolution in Philosophy* (London, Macmillan, 1960), p. 8.

Chapter 5
Geometry

1 M. Tiles, *Mathematics and the Image of Reason* (London, Routledge, 1991), p. 89.
2 S.W. Hawking, *A Brief History of Time* (London, Bantam Press, 1988), pp. 164–5.
3 G. Frege, *Posthumous Writings*, Vol. 1, translated by P. Long, R. White and R. Hargreaves (London, Blackwell, 1979), p. 169.
4 D. Hilbert, *Philosophy of Mathematics*, ed by E.P. Benacerraf and H. Putnan (Cambridge, Cambridge University Press, 1983), p. 186.
5 I. Kant, *Critique of Pure Reason*, translated by J.M.D. Meiklejohn (London, J.M. Dent, 1934), p. 260.
6 Hawking, *Brief History of Time*, pp. 7–8.
7 B. Russell, 'Introduction' to *Wittgenstein's Tractatus Logico-Philosophicus*, translated by D. F. Pears and B. F. McGuinness (London, Routledge and Kegan Paul, 1961), p. xvii.
8 Ibid., p. xvi.
9 M. Dummett, *Frege – Philosophy of Mathematics* (London, Duckworth, 1991), p. 321.
10 Kant, *Critique*, p. 12.
11 Tiles, *Mathematics and Image of Reason*, pp.126–7.

Chapter 6
Measurement and numbers

1 B. Orchard (ed.), *A Catholic Commentary on Holy Scripture* (Edinburgh, Thomas Nelson, 1953), p. 110.
2 O.A.W. Dilke *Mathematics and Measurement* (London, British Museum Press, 1987).
3 M . Dummett, *Frege – Philosophy of Mathematics* (London, Duckworth, (1991), p. 307.
4 P. Kenneth Seidelmann (ed.), *Explanatory Supplement to the Astronomical*

Almanac (Mill Valley, California, University Science Books, 1992).

5 H.S. Jones, *General Astronomy* 2nd edn (London, Edward Arnold, 1934), p. 12.

6 *Explanatory Supplement to the Astronomical Ephemeris and American Ephemeris and Nautical Almanac* (London, H.M. Stationery Office 1961), p. 68.

7 E.T. Whittaker, 'Spin in the Universe', reprint from *Year Book of the Royal Society of Edinburgh* (Edinburgh, Oliver and Boyd, 1945), pp. 1–9.

8 Seidelmann, *Explanatory Supplement*, p. 262, section 4.45.

9 S. O'Donnell, *William Rowan Hamilton* (Dublin, Boole Press, 1983), pp. 145–6.

10 W.R. Hamilton, *The Mathematical Papers of Sir William Rowan Hamilton* (Cambridge, Cambridge University Press, 1967), Vol. 3, p. 111.

11 Ibid., p. 152.

12 M. Crowe, *A History of Vector Analysis* (Paris, London, University of Notre Dame Press, 1967), p. 28.

13 B.L. Van der Waerden, 'Hamilton's Discovery of Quaternions', *Mathematical Magazine*, Vol. 49, No. 5, November 1976, pp. 227–34.

14 Ibid., p. 230.

15 W.R. Hamilton, *The Mathematical Papers of Sir William Rowan Hamilton* (Cambridge, Cambridge University Press, 1967), Vol. 3, p. 358.

16 Ibid., p. 152.

17 P.G. Tait, *An Elementary Treatise on Quaternions* (Oxford, 1867).

Chapter 7
Quaternions versus vector analysis

1 Michael J. Crowe, *A History of Vector Analysis* (Paris, London, University of Notre Dame Press, 1967), p. v.

2 Reginald J. Stephenson, 'Development of Vector Analysis from Quaternions', *American Journal of Physics* (1966), Vol. 34, p. 194.

3 W.R. Hamilton, *The Mathematical Papers of Sir William Rowan Hamilton* (Cambridge, Cambridge University Press, 1967), Vol. 3, p. 236.

4 Ibid., p. 147.

5 Cornelius Lanczos, 'William Rowan Hamilton – An Appreciation', *American Scientist* (1967), 55.2.

6 L.E. Dickson, 'On Quaternions and Their Generalization and the History of the Eight Square Theorem', *Annals of Mathematics*, 2nd series (Lancaster and Princeton, 1918–19), Vol. 20, p. 159.

7 Oliver Heavyside (1925), quoted from Michael Crowe, *A History of Vector Analysis* (New York, Dover Publications, 1994), p. 171.

8 C.G. Knott (1892), quoted from Crowe, *History of Vector Analysis* p. 202.

9 Ibid., p. 203.

10 Thomas L. Hankins, *Sir William Rowan Hamilton* (London, Baltimore,

Johns Hopkins University Press, 1980), p. 316.
11 C. Lanczos, 'Sir William Rowan Hamilton – An Appreciation', *University Review of the National University of Ireland* (1967), Vol. IV, No. 2, p. 162.
12 Hamilton, *Mathematical Papers* Vol. 3, pp. 153–4 footnote.
13 Parry Moon and Domina Spencer, *Vectors* (Princeton, New Jersey, D. Van Nostrand, 1965).
14 W.R. Hamilton quoted from Sean O'Donnell, *William Rowan Hamilton* (Dublin, Boole Press, 1983), p. 192.
15 Hamilton, *Mathematical Papers*, Vol. 3, p. 226.
16 Ibid., p. 361.
17 Ibid., p. 381.
18 Ibid., pp. 643–4.

Chapter 8
The unification of physics

1 N. Curran, *The Logical Universe: The Real Universe* (Aldershot, Avebury, 1994), p. 50.
2 J.D. Barrow, *The World Within the World* (Oxford, Oxford University Press, 1990), p. 115.
3 P. Davies, *God and the New Physics* (London, Penguin Books, 1988), p. viii.
4 G.J. Whitrow, *The Natural Philosophy of Time*, 2nd edn (Oxford, Clarendon Press, 1980), pp. 20–21.
5 S. Hawking, *A Brief History of Time* (London, Bantam Press, 1988), p. 145.
6 I. Stewart, *From Here to Infinity* (Oxford, Oxford University Press, 1996), p. 235.
7 Herman Minkowski (1907), quoted from Abraham Pais, *Subtle is the Lord – The Science and Life of Albert Einstein* (Oxford, Oxford University Press, 1983), pp. 151–2.
8 Ibid., p. 152.
9 A. Einstein, *The Meaning of Relativity* (London, Chapman and Hall, 1991), p. 37.
10 Whitrow, *Natural Philosophy of Time*, pp. 3–4.
11 Paul Davies, *About Time – Einstein's Unfinished Revolution* (New York, Simon and Schuster, 1995), p. 17.
12 Ibid., p. 278.
13 Ibid., p. 283.
14 Barrow, *The World Within the World*, p. 100.
15 E.T. Whittaker, 'Spin in the Universe', reprint from *Year Book of the Royal Society of Edinburgh* (Edinburgh, Oliver and Boyd, 1945), p. 7.
16 A. Pais, *Subtle is the Lord – The Science and Life of Albert Einstein*

(Oxford, Oxford University Press, 1983), p. 282.

17 Ibid., p. 243.

18 Barrow, *The World Within the World*, pp. 192–3.

19 W.R. Hamilton, *The Mathematical Papers of Sir William Rowan Hamilton* (Cambridge, Cambridge University Press, 1967), Vol. 3, p. 133, footnote.

20 Roger Penrose, *Shadows of the Mind* (Oxford, Oxford University Press, 1994), p. 384.

21 Pais, *Subtle is the Lord*, p. 210.

22 E. Schrödinger, *Scripta Mathematica* (1945), Vol. 2, p. 82.

23 P.A.M. Dirac, *The Principles of Quantum Mechanics*, 4th edn (Oxford, Clarendon Press, 1981), p. 84.

24 Barrow, *The World Within the World*, p. 147.

25 Dirac, *Principles of Quantum Mechanics*, p. 25.

26 E.T. Whittaker, 'The New Algebras and Their Significance for Physics and Philosophy', reprint from *Year Book of the Royal Society of Edinburgh* (Edinburgh, Oliver and Boyd, 1944), p. 9.

27 Davies, *About Time*, pp. 178–9.

28 Ibid., p. 179.

29 Stephen Hawking and Roger Penrose, *The Nature of Space and Time* (Princeton, New Jersey, Princeton University Press, 1996), p. 75.

30 Ibid., p. 76.

31 Curran, *The Logical Universe*, pp. 61–2.

32 Lewis Wolpert, *The Unnatural Nature of Science* (London, Faber & Faber, 1992), p. 106.

33 Ibid., p.108.

34 Steven Weinberg, *Dreams of a Final Theory* (London, Hutchinson Radius, 1993), p. 134.

35 James Jeans, *Physics and Philosophy* (Cambridge, Cambridge University Press, 1942), p. 47.

36 Ibid., p. 157.

37 Werner Heisenberg, *Physics and Philosophy* (London, Allen and Unwin Ltd., 1958), p. 52.

38 John Barrow, *Pi in the Sky* (London, Penguin Books, 1993), p. viii.

39 Ibid., p. 296.

40 E. Husserl, 'On the Concept of Number', in *Husserl – Shorter Works,* ed. by McCormick and Ellison (Paris, University of Notre Dame Press, 1981), pp. 95–6.

41 Ibid., p. 103.

42 Simon L. Altman, *Rotations Quaternions and Double Groups* (Oxford, Clarendon Press, 1986), p. 23.

43 J.C. Maxwell (1871), quoted from Michael Crowe, *A History of Vector Analysis* (New York, Dover Publications, 1994), p. 131.

44 *The Authorised Daily Prayer Book of the United Hebrew Congregations* (Cambridge, The Press Syndicate of the University of Cambridge, 1992),

p. 154.

45 John Paul II, *Physics, Philosophy and Theology*, ed. by R.J. Russell, W.R. Stoeger, SJ and G.V. Coyne, SJ, Vatican Observatory, Vatican City State (1988), P.M. 12.

46 Wolpert, *The Unnatural Nature of Science*, p. 144.

47 Ibid., pp. 145–6.

48 Herman Bondi, *The Times*, 20 May 1991.

49 Richard Dawkins, *Independent*, 12 August 1993.

50 Weinberg, *Dreams of a Final Theory*, p. 193.

51 John Macquarrie, *Heidegger and Christianity* (London, SCM Press, 1994), p. 7.

52 Edmund Whittaker, *Space and Spirit* (London, Thomas Nelson, 1946), p. 120.

53 St Augustine, *The City of God* (London, J.M. Dent, 1945), Vol. I. p. 317.

54 Joseph Ratzinger, *In the Beginning*, translated by B. Ramsey O.P. (Huntington, Indiana, Our Sunday Visitor, 1990).

55 John Polkinghorne, *Science and Christian Belief* (London, SPCK, 1994), p. 73.

56 Curran, *The Logical Universe*, p. 135.

57 *Catechism of the Catholic Church* (London, Geoffrey Chapman), para 293, p. 69.

58 Wolpert, *The Unnatural Nature of Science*, pp. 145–6.

59 Peter Atkins, from *Manchester Evening News*, 13 September 1996, p. 8.

60 Peter Atkins, *Creation Revisited* (London, Penguin Books, 1994), p. vii.

61 Ibid., p. 99.

Bibliography

Altman, Simon L. (1986), *Rotations, Quaternions and Double Groups*, Clarendon Press: Oxford.

Anscombe, G.E.M. (1959), *An Introduction to Wittgenstein's Tractatus*, Hutchinson University Library: London.

Aquinas, St Thomas (1945), *Commentary on Aristotle's Physics*, translated by James A. McWilliams S.J. Catholic University of America: Washington.

Atkins, Peter (1994), *Creation Revisited*, Penguin Books: London.

Atkins, Peter (1996), from *Manchester Evening News*, 13 September.

Ayer, A.J. (1946), *Language, Truth and Logic*, Victor Gollancz: London.

Ayer, A.J. (1973), *The Central Questions of Philosophy*, Penguin Books: London.

Barrow, John D. (1990), *The World Within the World*. Oxford University Press: Oxford.

Barrow, John D. (1993), *Pi in the Sky*, Penguin Books: London.

Bell, David (1990), *Husserl*, Routledge: London.

Crowe, M. (1967), *A History of Vector Analysis*, University of Notre Dame Press: Notre Dame, London.

Crowe, Michael J. (1994), *A History of Vector Analysis*, Dover Publications: New York.

Curran, N. (1994), *The Logical Universe: The Real Universe*, Avebury: Aldershot and Brookfield USA.

Davies, P. (1988), *God and the New Physics*, Penguin Books: London.

Davies, Paul (1995), *About Time – Einstein's Unfinished Revolution*, Simon and Schuster: New York.

Dawkins, Richard (1993), from *Independent*, 12 August.

Dickson, L.E. (1918–19), *Annals of Mathematics*, 2nd series, Vol. 20, Lancaster and Princeton.

Dilke, O.A.W. (1987), *Mathematics and Measurement*, British Museum Press: London.

Dirac, P.A.M. (1981), *The Principles of Quantum Mechanics*, 4th edn, Clarendon Press: Oxford.

Dummett, M. (1991), *Frege – Philosophy of Mathematics*, Duckworth: London.

Einstein, A. (1944), *Relativity: The Special and General Theory*, Methuen: London.

Einstein, A. (1991), *The Meaning of Relativity*, Chapman and Hall: London.

Frege, G. (1884), *The Foundations of Arithmetic*, translated by J.L. Austin, Blackwell: Oxford.

Frege, G. (1960), *Translations from the philosophical writings of Gottlob Frege*, ed. by P. Geach and M. Black, Blackwell: Oxford.

Frege, G. (1979), *Posthumous Writings, Vol. 1*, translated by P. Long, R. White and R. Hargreaves, Blackwell: London.

Hamilton, W.R. (1967), *The Mathematical Papers of Sir William Rowan Hamilton*, Vol. 3, Cambridge University Press: Cambridge.

Hamilton W.R. (1846), from Sean O'Donnell (1983), *William Rowan Hamilton*, Boole Press: Dublin.

Hankins, T. L. (1980), *Sir William Rowan Hamilton*, Johns Hopkins University Press: Baltimore.

Hawking, S.W. (1988), *A Brief History of Time*, Bantam Press: London.

Hawking, Stephen and Penrose, Roger (1996), *The Nature of Space and Time*, Princeton University Press, Princeton: New Jersey.

Heavyside, Oliver (1925), quoted from Michael Crowe (1994), *A History of Vector Analysis*, Dover Publications: New York.

Heidegger, M. (1962), *Being and Time*, translated by J. Macquarrie and E. Robinson, SCM Press: London.

Heisenberg, Werner (1958), *Physics and Philosophy*, Allen and Unwin Ltd: London.

Herman, Bondi (1991), *The Times*, 20 May.

Hilbert, D. (1983), *Philosophy of Mathematics*, ed. by E.P. Benacerraf and H. Putnan, Cambridge University Press: Cambridge.

Husserl, E. (1887), 'On the Concept of Number', in McCormick & Ellison (eds) (1981), *Husserl – Shorter Works*, University of Notre Dame Press: Notre Dame.

Husserl, E. (1891), *Philosophie der Arithmetic*, Husserliana Vol. 12, Nijhoff: The Hague.

Husserl, E. (1931), *Ideas – General Introduction to Pure Phenomenology*, translated by W.R. Boyce Gibson, George Allen & Unwin: London.

Husserl, E. (1970), *Logical Investigations* Vol. 1, translated by J.N. Findlay, Routledge & Kegan Paul: London.

Jeans, James (1942), *Physics and Philosophy*, Cambridge University Press: Cambridge.

John Paul II (1988), *Physics, Philosophy and Theology*, ed. by R.J. Russell, W.R. Stoeger, S.J. and G.V. Coyne, S.J, Vatican Observatory: Vatican City State, P.M. 12.

Jones, H.S. (1934), *General Astronomy*, 2nd edn, Edward Arnold: London.

Kant, I. (1783–1953), *Prolegomena to any Future Metaphysics*, translated by Peter G. Lucas, Manchester University Press: Manchester.

Kant, I. (1934), *The Critique of Pure Reason*, translated by J.M.D. Meiklejohn, J.M. Dent: London.

Kneale, W, and M. (1962), *The Development of Logic*, Clarendon Press: Oxford.

Lanczos, C. (1967), 'William Rowan Hamilton – An Appreciation', *University Review of the National University of Ireland*, Vol. IV, No. 2.

Lanczos, C. (1967), 'William Rowan Hamilton – An Appreciation', *American Scientist*, 55.2.

Macquarrie, John (1994), *Heidegger and Christianity*, SCM Press: London.

Maxwell, J.C. (1871), from Michael Crowe (1994), *A History of Vector Analysis*, Dover Publications: New York.

Minkowski, Herman (1907), quoted from Abraham Pais (1983), *Subtle is the Lord – The Science and Life of Albert Einstein*, Oxford University Press: Oxford.

Moon, Parry and Spencer, Domina (1965), *Vectors*, D. Van Nostrand: Princeton, New Jersey.

Newton-Smith, W.H. (1980), *The Structure of Time*, Routledge and Kegan Paul: London.

O'Donnell, S. (1983), *William Rowan Hamilton*, Boole Press: Dublin.

Orchard, B. (ed.) (1953), *A Catholic Commentary on Holy Scripture*, Thomas Nelson: Edinburgh.

Pais, A. (1983), *Subtle is the Lord – The Science and Life of Albert Einstein*, Oxford University Press: Oxford.

Passmore, J. (1954), *A Hundred Years of Philosophy*, Duckworth: London.

Penrose, R. (1989), *The Emperor's New Mind*, Oxford University Press: Oxford.

Penrose, Roger (1994), *Shadows of the Mind*, Oxford University Press: Oxford.

Polkinghorne, John (1994), *Science and Christian Belief*, SPCK: London.

Ratzinger, Joseph (1990), *In the Beginning*, translated by B. Ramsey O.P., Our Sunday Visitor: Huntington, Indiana.

Russell, B. (1914), *Our Knowledge of the External World*, Open Court Publishing Company: Chicago, London.

Russell, B. (1919), *Introduction to Mathematical Philosophy*, George Allen and Unwin: London.

Russell, B. (1961), Introduction to *Wittgenstein's Tractatus Logico-*

Philosophicus, translated by D.F. Pears and B.F. McGuinness, Routledge and Kegan Paul: London.

Ryle, G. (1960), *The Revolution in Philosophy*, Macmillan & Co. Ltd: London.

Schrödinger, E, (1945), *Scripta Mathematica, Vol. 2*.

Seidelmann, P. Kenneth (ed.) (1992), *Explanatory Supplement to the Astronomical Almanac*, University Science Books: Mill Valley, California.

St Augustine (1945), *The City of God, Vol. I*, J.M. Dent: London.

Stebbing, S. (1946), *A Modern Introduction to Logic*, Methuen: London.

Stephenson, Reginald J. (1966), 'Development of Vector Analysis from Quaternions', *American Journal of Physics*, Vol. 34.

Stewart, I. (1996), *From Here to Infinity*, Oxford University Press: Oxford.

Tait, P.G. (1867), *An Elementary Treatise on Quaternions*, Oxford.

Temple, G. (1981), *100 Years of Mathematics*, Duckworth: London.

Tiles, M. (1991), *Mathematics and the Image of Reason*, Routledge: London.

Van Der Waerden, B.L. (1976), *Mathematical Magazine*, Vol. 49, No. 5, November.

Weinberg, Steven (1993), *Dreams of a Final Theory*, Hutchinson Radius: London.

Whitrow, G.J. (1961), *The Natural Philosophy of Time*, Thomas Nelson: London.

Whitrow, G.J. (1980), *The Natural Philosophy of Time*, 2nd edn, Clarendon Press: Oxford.

Whittaker, E.T. (1940), 'The Hamiltonian Revival', *The Mathematical Gazette*, Vol. 24, No. 260.

Whittaker, E.T. (1943), 'The New Algebras and Their Significance for Physics and Philosophy', reprint from *Year Book of Royal Society of Edinburgh* (1944), Oliver and Boyd: Edinburgh.

Whittaker, E.T. (1944), 'The Sequence of Ideas in the Discovery of Quaternions', *Pro. Royal Irish Academy*, Vol. 50A, No. 6.

Whittaker, E.T. (1944), 'Spin In The Universe', reprint from *Year Book of the Royal Society of Edinburgh* (1945), Oliver and Boyd: Edinburgh and London.

Whittaker, Edmund (1946), *Space and Spirit*, Thomas Nelson: London.

Wittgenstein, L. (1961), *Tractatus Logico-Philosophicus*, translated by D.F. Pears and B.F. McGuinness, Routledge & Kegan Paul: London.

Wolpert, Lewis (1992), *The Unnatural Nature of Science*, Faber & Faber: London.

Catechism of the Catholic Church (1994), Chapman Geoffrey: London.

Explanatory Supplement (1961) to the Astronomical Ephemeris and American Ephemeris and Nautical Almanac (1961), H.M. Stationery Office: London.

The Authorised Daily Prayer Book of the United Hebrew Congregations (1992), The Press Syndicate of the University of Cambridge: Cambridge.

Index

Abelard, Peter: *Sic et Non* 7, 172
Altman, Simon 175
analytical a priori judgements (Kant)
    25, 26–7, 87–8
angle, measurement by 95
anisotropic, 142, 152
Anscombe, Elizabeth 6
Anselm, St 91
antinomy 81–4
apodeictic judgements 4, 76
Aquinas, St Thomas 68–9, 91, 178,
    180, 182
    Summa Theologica 8
Archimedes 146
Aristotelian system of the cosmos 14
Aristotle 6, 61, 76, 85, 96, 98, 102,
    103, 182
    demonstrative premise (apodeiktike
      protasis) 4, 6
    Physics 68
    Topics 7
arithmogram 123
arrow of time (time direction;
    Zeitrichtung) 10, 63, 64–70,
    139–42
Aspect, Alain 160
associative law of addition 10

atheism 101, 178, 180–2, 184
Atkins, Professor Peter 188, 189
atomic time 102, 104
Augustine, St 83, 182
axiomatic set theory 21–9
    application of mathematiucs 26–7
    branches of mathematics 27–8
    cardinal numbers 21
    cardinal numbers and ordinal
      numbers 22–3
    cardinal numbers have no direct
      references 25
    cardinal sets 21
    commutative law 24
    concept of counting 23–4
    concept of meaning in mathematics
      26
    concept of value-ranges 24–5
    formal logic 25–6
    one-to-one correspondence 21–2
    problem of zero and one 22
axioms 4, 14, 18
Ayer, Alfred 46, 47, 172
    Language, Truth and Logic 13,
      26–7, 47, 72

Barrow, John 89, 160–1

Pi in the Sky 173
World Within the World, The 137,
147, 150
Bell, David: *Philosophy of Arithmetic*
28–9
Benacerraf, Paul 24, 47
Big Bang theory of cosmology 139,
166–9
Bohr 137, 159
theory of the atom 158
Bondi, Herman 167, 179, 182
Boole's symbolic logic 43
Bosanquet 100
Bradley 69, 100

Cantor 16, 21, 78
theory of transfinite numbers 79
cardinal numbers 13
Cayley, Arthur 7, 43, 50, 133, 162
algebra of dimension 8 124, 128
geometry of *n*-dimensions 115
Celsius scale of temperature 63, 95
coherence theory 86
commutative algebra 7, 8, 10
law of addition 10
law of multiplication 3, 7, 8, 24
complex numbers 38–42, 46, 52
conservation laws 137
Conway, Professor A.W. 49, 111
coordinated universal time (UTC)
104–5
Copernican Revolution 14, 87, 103,
105–8, 148, 152
Copernicus 98, 179
Corpus Agrimensorum 97
cosmology 99, 166–9
Ptolemaic system of 14, 105
Coyne, Fr. Vincent 178
Crowe, Michael: *History of Vector
Analysis, A* 114, 120, 124, 128,
134
cyclical measure 95

Davies, Paul 139, 147
About Time 146, 153, 162
Dawkins, Richard 101, 180
de Sitter 103
declarative sentence 5, 10

dialectical logic 7, 10, 15, 52, 72
Dickson, L.E. 124
Dilke, O.A.W.: *Mathematics and
Measurement* 97
Dilthey 98
Dirac, Paul 43, 50, 156, 159
equation 49
Principles of Quantum Mechanics
161
dogmas 179
Doppler effect 80, 166
Dummett, Michael 15, 16, 27–8, 30,
32, 73, 85
Frege – Philosophy of Mathematics
9, 27, 101
dynamical time 102, 104, 105

Einstein 123, 146, 150, 153, 171
theory of relativity 48, 99, 107, 165
general theory of relativity
(theory of gravitation) 90,
137, 154, 155–7
special theory of relativity 136,
142–7
elliptical geometry 76, 79, 155
ephemeris time 102, 103, 107, 165
equality, theory of 15
equations of motion 7
Euclidean geometry 8, 28, 73–7, 93–4
universe as 78–81
expansion of the universe 80, 166–9

falsifiability, Popper's theory of 26
fluxions 33
formal logic 4, 7, 10, 23–4, 52, 72
Foucault 148–9
pendulum 106, 150
Frege 16, 33, 59, 61
Basic Laws of Arithmetic 27
Foundations of Arithmetics 7, 27,
30, 41, 69
Function and Begriff 8
Grundgesetze 12, 30, 54
Grundlagen 9, 10, 25
on cardinal numbers 98, 99
On Meaning and Reference 7, 30, 62
on non-Euclidean geometry 76
on real numbers 30–2

principle of value-ranges 46, 67
theory of judgement 1–15
theory of truth-functions 26
Uber Sinn und Bedeutung 1, 17–20
Frobenius, G. 128

Gadamer, Hans Georg 98
Gale 149
Galileo 98, 107, 146, 148, 179
Gauss 121
Geisteswissenschaften 98, 99, 177
geometry, definition 73
Gibbs, Josiah Willard
    dyadics 43
    Elements of Vector Analysis 124
    vector analysis 121, 124–35
God, existence or non-existence 13,
    91–2, 177–90
Gödel 16
Gold 167, 182
grammarithm 49, 112, 113, 114, 123
Grassmann, Professor H:
    Ausdehnungslehre (Theory of
    Extension) 43, 50, 116, 125, 127,
    128
Graves 114
gravitation, theory of 75–6, 80–1, 90,
    136
    laws for 138
Green 121
Grimes, Andrew 189
Grossmann, Marcel 150, 156, 171
gyrocompass 150
gyroscope 106, 112, 133, 150
gyroscopic inertia 150

Hamilton, Sir William Rowan 32–4,
    42, 47, 55–72, 61, 69, 128, 140,
    142, 157, 176, 190
    *Conjugate Functions or Algebraic
    Couples* 39
    Elements of Quaternions 32, 48, 59,
    124
    grammarithm 49, 112, 113, 114, 123
    Lectures on Quaternions 32, 33, 39,
    55, 58, 59, 61, 122, 124
    Mathematical Papers 55, 133
    On a General Method in Dynamics

32, 158
on algebra 56
*On Algebra as the Science of Pure
    Time* 39, 55, 73
on imaginary numbers 58–9, 60–1
on time 33–4, 36, 57–9, 61
quaternions and spin 110–19
theory of wave mechanisms 159
Hankel, Herman: *Vorlesungen über
    die Complexen Zahlen 1867* 69
Hankins, Thomas 59, 126, 127
Hawking, Stephen 63, 75, 83, 166,
    167, 188
    Brief History of Time 140
Heavyside, Oliver 125, 128, 129, 130,
    134
    Electromagnetic Theory 125
Hebrew measures 97
Hegel 86, 100
Heidegger 181, 182
    Being and Time 4, 24, 96, 98
Heisenberg, Werner 137
    Physics and Philosophy 84, 170
    uncertainty principle 51, 159
heresy 179
Herschel 131
    theory time–space 131
Hesse, Mary: *Science and the Human
    Imagination* 45
Hilbert, David 14, 16, 26, 74, 78–9,
    173
    Philosophy of Mathematics 32, 47
Hilbert Space 51, 67
Hipparchus 107
Hoyle 167, 182
Hubble's theory of an expanding
    universe 166
Hume: *Treatise of Human Nature, A*
    98
Hurvitz, Adolph 128
Husserl 16, 21, 33, 61
    Ideas I 4, 18, 99
    Logical Investigations 2, 5
    on internal time-consciousness 101
    Phenomenology 98
    Philosophy of Arithmetic 25, 27,
    28–9, 69, 73, 174
    theory of intentionality 10

theory of time 28
hypercomplex numbers 49–54

imaginary numbers, Hamilton on
    58–9, 60–1
imprecision, concept of 51
intentionality 10
international atomic time (TAI) 104
International Earth Rotation Service
    (IERS) 108
intransitive counting 24

Jeans, Sir James: *Physics and*
    Philosophy 170
John Paul II, Pope 178
judgement, definition 1

Kant, I. 4, 9, 25, 61
    Critique of Pure Reason 18, 56
    first antinomy 81–4, 93
    on internal time-consciousness 101
    philosophy of mathematical physics
        87–92
        analytical a priori judgement 25,
            26–7, 87–8
        existence is not a predicate 90
        on ontological argument for
            existence of God 91–2
        on space 88
        on the Copernican Revolution
            88–90
        on time 88–9
    Prolegomena to any Future
        Metaphysics 9, 18
    synthetic a priori judgements 9, 18,
        25, 28, 56, 83, 86
Kelvin scale of temperature 63, 95,
    152
Klein, Felix 129
Kneales, W. and M.: *Development of*
    Logic, The 4, 6
Knott, Cargill Gilston 125–6, 128
Kung, Hans 183

Lagrange 33, 146
Lanczos, Cornelius 48, 113, 117, 123,
    124, 127
Lavoisier 146

laws of motion 78, 146
laws of nature 137–9, 163, 181
laws of quantum theory 138, 181
leap seconds 105
length, measurement of 96, 97
Levi-Civita 157
light, speed of 143, 155–6, 164
light cone 144
logic 16–20, 171–2
    formal 4, 7, 10, 23–4, 52, 72
logic of being 100
logical universe theory 94
Lorentz transformations 143
Lunar Laser-Ranging (LLR) 107

MacFarlane 126, 129
Mach, Ernest 149
Macquarrie, John 181–2
Maimonides, Moses: *Thirteen*
        Principles 178
matrix algebra 7, 25, 50, 162
Maxwell, James Clerk 121, 176
    equations 143
McTaggert 69
meaningless 13
measure numbers 95
Michelson 149
Minkowski 146, 171, 190
    space–time 144–5, 152, 153–4, 175
Moon, Parry 128
Moore 72
multidimensional geometry 115

Napier 33
Naturwissenschaft 98
Newton 33, 89, 99, 107, 148, 155, 160
    laws of motion 78, 146
    theory of gravitation 90, 107
Newton-Smith, W.H. 61, 62
    Structure of Time, The 83
noema 11
noematic experience 10
noesis 11
noetic experience 10, 11
non-commutative algebra 7, 8, 10, 28,
    66–7, 161
    n-dimensions 66
    one dimension of time 67

three dimensions 66
two dimensions 66–7
non-commutative multiplication 66
non-Euclidean geometry 8, 9, 28,
   73–7, 93–4
   universe as 78–81
non-locality, phenomenon of 160–1
nonsense 13
number, meaning of 12

O'Donnell, Sean 110, 113, 118
   William Rowan Hamilton 44
onto-logic 92, 100

Pais, Abraham 123
   Subtle is the Lord 155
Pauli 49
Peano 16
   axioms of number 22
Penrose, Roger 66, 153
   Emperor's New Mind, The 31, 63,
   159
picture theory (Wittgenstein) 6, 14
Pippard, Sir Brian 106
Planck, Max 137, 158
Planck's constant 51, 106, 158, 159
Plato 61, 182
   Timaeus 61
polar opposites 11
Polkinghorne, Reverend John 188
   Science and Christian Belief 183
Popper's theory of falsifiability 26
precession 107, 150
proof theory 4
proposition, definition 1
Ptolemaic system of cosmology 14, 105
Putnam, Hilary 47, 169

quantum mechanics 43
quantum theory 157–65
   laws for 138, 181
   mathematics of 161
   time and 162–5
quaternions, Hamilton's 7, 15, 32,
   42–9, 51, 54, 174–5
   spin and 110–19, 150–2
   vectors and 52, 121–4

radians 95
Ratzinger, Cardinal Joseph 182
real numbers 35–8
reality 172
red-shift 80–1, 166, 168, 169
relativity, general theory of 84, 94
religion, science and 177–90
Ricci 157
Rickert 98
Riemann's elliptic geometry 76, 155
Roman measures 97
Rosse, Lady 110, 119
rotation 107
Russell, Bertrand 16, 31, 84
   on complex numbers 41
   *Introduction to Mathematical
   Philosophy* 41
   on logical atomism 36, 86
   on ordinal and cardinal numbers 23
   *Our Knowledge of the External
   World* 69
   on time 69–70
Ryle, Gilbert, 72
   Revolution in Philosophy, The 5

Saccheri, G.: *Euclides ab omni naevo
   vindicatus* 76
Satellite Laser-Ranging (SLR) 107
scalar numbers 36–7, 56, 85, 95
Schrödinger 32, 137, 159, 165
sentence, definition 1
sidereal time 102
simultaneity, concept of 186
space
   finite vs infinite 78–9
   flat vs curved 78
   gravitation and 80–1
space–time, Minkowski's 144–5, 152,
   153–4, 175
spacelike vector 144
Spencer, Domina 128
Spencer Jones, Sir Harold 102, 103
spherical geometry space 76
spin 85, 105–6, 107, 108–19, 129–30,
   148–50, 160
   Hamilton's quaternions and 150–2
spin matrices 49
steady-state theory of the universe

167, 182
Stebbing, Susan 46
Stephenson, Reginald J. 121
Stewart, Ian: *From Here to Infinity*
    143, 154
Stoke 121
Sylvester 43
Synge, J.L. 157
synthetic a priori judgements 9, 18, 25,
    28, 56, 83, 86

Tait, Peter Guthrie 124
    *Elementary Treatise on
    Quaternions, An* 116, 125
Tarner lectures 51
tautologies 20
TDB 104
Temple, George: *100 Years of
    Mathematics* 31, 36, 118
tensor analysis 171
tensor calculus 157
terrestrial dynamical time (TDT) 104
Tiles, Mary 92
    *Mathematics and the Image of
    reason* 74
time
    Aristotle on 68
    arrow of 10, 63, 64–70, 139–42
    as reference point 63
    duration of 10
    dynamical 102, 104, 105
    Hamilton on 57
    measurement of 96, 97, 101, 102–5,
    165
    Russell on 69–70
    types of scale 102
    uniform 104
    universal 102
timelike vector 144
transfinite numbers, Cantor's theory of
    79
transitive counting 24
translation 105, 109, 148–9

uncertainty principle, Heisenberg's 51,
    159
uniform time 104
units of measure, standardisation of

96–7
universal time 102
universe
    expansion 80, 166–9
    single vs multiple 80
    translatory motion and rotation 81

validity of judgements, concept of 4
validity, notion (concept) of 4
value-range 8, 24–5, 46, 47
Van der Waerden, B.L. 114, 115
vectors 120–35
    concept of 41
    Hamilton's quaternions and 52,
    121–4
    rotation of 130
    triple algebra of 131
versor 41
Very Long Baseline Interferometry
    (VLBI) 107–8

weight, measurement of 96, 97
Weinberg, Steven: *Dreams of a Final
    Theory* 170, 181
Whitehead 16
Whitrow, G.J. 67
    Natural Philosophy of Time, The
    64, 79, 139, 146
Whittaker, Sir Edmund 42, 51, 67,
    106, 118, 119, 133, 149, 162,
    166, 186
    Space and Spirit 182
Wigner 170
Wilson, Edwin Bidwell 124
Windleband 98
Wittgenstein 5, 173
    Brown Book 12
    meaning of words 13
    on tautologies 20
    Philosophical Investigations 12
    picture theory 6, 14
    Tractatus 6, 36, 72, 84
Wolpert, Lewis 179, 182, 187, 188
    Unnatural Nature of Science, The
    169, 178
world line 144

Yost, Professor Don M. 113

Printed and bound by CPI Group (UK) Ltd, Croydon, CR0 4YY

21/10/2024

01777087-0003